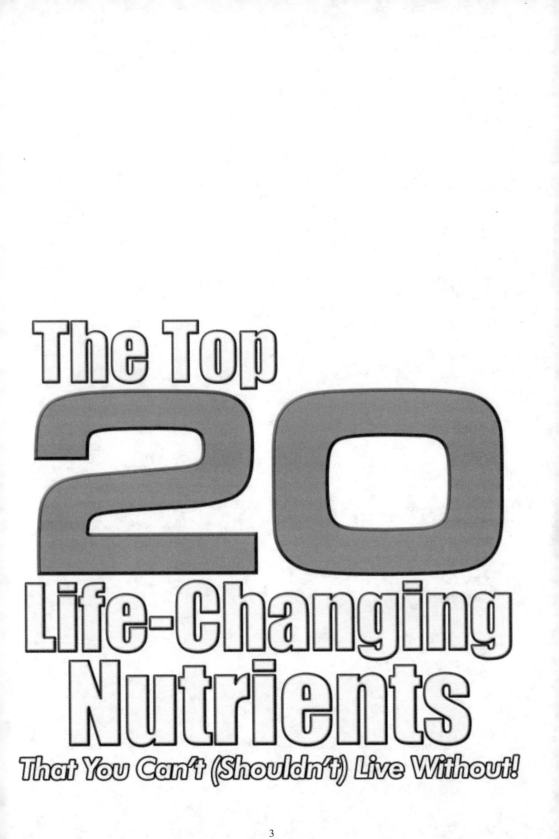

The Top 20 Life-Changing Nutrients

That You Can't (Shouldn't) Live Without!

The Top 20 Life-Changing Nutrients that You Can't (Shouldn't) Live Without!

Ward W. Bond, Ph.D.
with Peggy Nelson

The Top 20 Life-Changing Nutrients You Can't (Shouldn't) Live Without! and other Nutritional Living books are available at special quantity discounts.

For information contact:
800.620.9975

Other books by Ward W. Bond, Ph.D. (available at www.drwardbond.com) include:

Dr. Ward Bond's Vitamin, Mineral & Antioxidant Guide

Dr. Ward Bond's Natural Guide to Better Sex

Copyright © 2009 by Ward W. Bond
All rights reserved. No portion of this book may be reproduced or transmitted electronically without authorized consent of the author.

ISBN 978-0-982-1204-0-8
Library of Congress Cataloging-in-Publication Data

Printed in the United States of America

This book is dedicated to all those who desire life-changing optimal health

Table of Contents

Acknowledgements

I would like to take the opportunity to thank all the many people who were involved and participated in this book project. This book has been a goal of mine for many years and I am appreciative of the time, support and individual expertise of those who have made this book a reality. A special thanks goes to my co-writer Peggy Nelson who provided many long hours of technical support in writing and skillfully organizing the vast amount of information on many different nutrients compiled in this book into a concise and understandable format that brings the life-changing nutrients too well, life.

I am thankful to the professional guidance of Herschell Gordon Lewis who is not only a fellow colleague and health nut, but a precious family friend. Thank you Herschell for your overseeing this project and working with both Peggy and myself.

Special thanks to those who contributed to this book project with your incredible research and insights that have made many of the nutrients in this book truly life-changing. I would like to thank Dr. Douglas MacKay, ND; Mark Underwood, Kim Bright, Dr. David Dyer, Tony Lucchesi, Tom Bohager, Tom Vonderbrink, and Annie Eng for their contributions to the research of this book.

To my brother, Donald Bond for his talent in the graphic design of the book cover and getting the manuscript ready for publishing.

Last of all, I would like to acknowledge the support and encourage of my beautiful wife, Michelle, who with her love and inspiration has brought greater meaning and purpose to my life. To my children whom I love very much, Sterling and Madison for enduring the countless days, hours and minutes of getting this book done.

Foolish the doctor who despises the knowledge acquired by the ancients.
~ Hippocrates

Dear fellow reader,
I was inspired to write this book when I realized just how much marketing hype there is in today's natural health arena – so much so that it falls on deaf ears, and that's alarming. I realized it was what it was – hype – no substance. The research had been overshadowed.

What I found was 20 nutrients that would make a positive, dramatic impact your health and mine – with the research to back it up.

Medical research, nutritional research, and yes, the uses of nutrients throughout the centuries and from a multitude of cultures – I wanted to prove that excellent health is attainable and right now.

I believe in truth. This book contains truths about newly discovered nutrients such as Aequorin, which improves the lives of those who suffer from mental decline. The nutrient Ribose, (which we're born) improves the lives of those suffering with congestive heart failure, and fibromyalgia. It even improves the recovery time of athletes. The ancient uses of Maca, Maqui, and Lion's Mane give us a long history of the past and promises for a healthy future. When ancient medicinal nutrients meet the rich research of today, we have validity that our ancestors knew a lot of what we've lost in modern medicine.

My hope is that you can come away from this book with life-changing nutrients. My wish is that you become empowered in your own right for the responsibility of your own health. No matter your age. We can overcome disease even when medical research says we can't. Even when it ignores the very nutrients created for our bodies to extend life. Cancer, Alzheimer's, heart disease can all be diseases of the past.

These 20 nutrients are the first set of nutrients that are simple, extraordinarily effective, and life-changing. The researchers should be commended for spending countless hours, and years of clinical testing and more clinical testing, to prove to the world what Mother Nature provides us is sound. Natural medicinal nutrients have always been here for us to benefit from.

"By the river on its bank, on one side and on the other, will grow all kinds of trees for food. Their leaves will not wither and their fruit will not fail. They will bear every month because their water flows from the sanctuary, and their fruit will be for food and their leaves for healing.

New American Standard Bible

CHAPTER ONE

Aequorin

Aequorin
Getting old doesn't have to be a bummer

We all fear the process of getting old—not being able to do what we could when we were young … or even five years ago.

Those signs and symptoms of aging are challenging (if not debilitating):

- Stiffness and sore muscles
- Loss of energy and endurance
- Weakness
- Confusion and uncertainty
- Forgetfulness
- Worries about medical bills, or long-term care insurance

But the worst of all is we face the possibility of normal aging developing into a devastating illness like Alzheimer's disease.

Disease and Aging
Losing independence is one of the greatest fears people have in their "senior" years. The final stages of Alzheimer's inexorably strip victims of their memories, dignity, and eventually their lives. It's not an easy way to go.

When does it start? Physicians and researchers are beginning to think that early lapses in short-term memory or fleeting moments of confusion an individual experiences in their 40s and 50s, quickly attributed to stress or not getting enough sleep, could actually be the earliest stages of Alzheimer's disease.

Some 26.6 million people worldwide were living with the disease in 2006. Predictions are that by 2050 the number suffering from Alzheimer's disease will leap to more than 100 million, meaning 1 in 85 persons worldwide will be fighting this crippling illness. More than 40 percent of those individuals will be in late-stage Alzheimer's, which requires a very high level of personalized care.

Other frightening neurological disorders are striking aging Americans in increasing numbers. Parkinson's disease, multiple sclerosis, amyotrophic lateral sclerosis (ALS), Pick's disease, and stroke all are progressive in nature and impossible to treat effectively; they create huge amounts of emotional and physical trauma and wreck the victim's quality of life. Some 15 million people in the U.S. suffer from serious neurodegenerative disorders, and thousands more are diagnosed every year, as baby boomers grow older.

Soaring costs and a ray of hope

The cost of health care also continues to spiral out of control. (Unsurprisingly, older Americans have higher health-care costs.)

The average amount spent by Medicare on people with dementia (largely Alzheimer's) is almost three times more than the amount Medicare spends on other medical problems -- $13,207 versus $4,454 per year. Much of this money is devoted to hospital and nursing-home care. (One reason these costs are so high is that skilled nursing-home care is at least ten times more expensive for patients with dementia.)

Long-term care was not a thought 20 or 30 years ago. Due to Americans living longer and receiving better medical care, combined with the huge increase in lengthy debilitating conditions like Alzheimer's, long-term care policies have become increasingly expensive, beyond the ability of many aging Americans to afford.

In the United States alone, nearly $2 billion is spent every year on therapeutics for Alzheimer's disease. Add France, Germany, Italy, Spain, the United Kingdom, and Japan, and that number jumps to almost $4 billion per year. Despite these incredible sales figures and the collective hope for positive outcomes, existing medicines are woefully ineffective against Alzheimer's and other neurodegenerative diseases.

What can we do?

The standard approach in medicine is treating the symptoms, not the underlying causes. However—thankfully—we can treat the cause and the symptoms with a substance called Aequorin, available commercially as a product called Prevagen™.

The Answer: Aequorin, the Calcium Regulator

You may not have known that calcium is the most abundant mineral in our body and influences many aspects of our general health including brain cell function, bone formation, blood clotting, and wound healing.

Many of those terrible conditions can be linked to calcium imbalances in the body, which may result from reduced numbers of calcium-binding proteins. This depletion is thought to be a result of aging or the disease process. The job of this incredible, hard-working compound is to "lock up" excess calcium in the bloodstream and tissue, by protecting the nervous system from the negative effects of too much calcium. This maximizes cellular health by protecting the brain, cognitive function, memory, and neuronal connectivity. Using Aequorin is a great way to regulate calcium in our bodies, whether we already suffer from calcium-related illnesses or simply want to take a proactive approach to maintain the best possible health.

The Role of Calcium in Aging

Most Americans know how important calcium is for healthy bones and teeth. But the role calcium plays goes far beyond the skeleton. Calcium is essential for brain cell health and the efficient transmission of messages throughout the nervous system. It's also important for keeping genes and cells healthy, active, and supple. But if there is too much calcium in our neurons, critical chemical reactions start to bog down. Over time, this may lead to earlier onset of the physical changes associated with aging, as well as serious afflictions such as Alzheimer's.

As we age, our bodies produce fewer and fewer important proteins, resulting in too much ionic calcium floating through our bloodstream and tissues. This extra calcium is particularly troublesome for aging neurons. A number of studies suggest that when these neurons are activated, too much calcium interferes with the cell reactions and causes "misfiring" throughout the nervous system—especially in brain regions tied to memory.

> *A decrease in the number of calcium-binding proteins in our bodies can result in too much calcium within our cells, which accelerates the aging process, chronic or acute inflammation, and the onset of serious neurological diseases.*

Over the past fifteen years, scientists have established that a breakdown in regulating calcium is a major factor in the development of aging-related learning and memory problems. Studies suggest that loss of important proteins with advancing age may leave neurons vulnerable to even moderate increases in the amount of intracellular calcium. The relationship between calcium, neuron degeneration, calcium-binding proteins, and aging suggests that replenishing these proteins in the neurons, through supplementation, will slow the effects of aging.

Calcium's Link to Disease

With most major neurodegenerative diseases, there is an excess of unregulated calcium in the areas that are afflicted, such as the brain. As these diseases progress and the calcium "homeostasis" (stable condition) goes awry, the concentration of free calcium ions in the nervous system increases. The body steadily loses its ability to control how this calcium is stored and used. These free-roaming excess calcium ions start to wreak havoc on neurons. The unregulated calcium triggers damaging cellular events that impair and eventually kill the neurons. Increased total calcium levels, as well as reductions in key calcium-binding proteins, have been found in patients with Alzheimer's, Huntington's, and Parkinson's diseases.

So what can we conclude?

Calcium-binding proteins serve an important role in protecting neurons from calcium overload and keeping the cellular circuitry firing properly. The easiest way to replenish the calcium-binding proteins that we lose as we age is with Prevagen.

Protecting Brain Cells with Aequorin

Until Aequorin, there were no effective therapeutics for treating the problem of excess calcium ions and the loss of calcium-binding proteins. Aequorin, marketed as Prevagen, is the first supplement to fight the aging process by replenishing these powerful proteins, which protect our cells from unhealthy amounts of intracellular calcium.

Even in healthy individuals, the mere process of aging causes much of our brain cell activity to falter and slow down. The natural wear and tear on brain cells as we age, and their ability to function at optimal levels, depends in part on having the proper balance of calcium.

Normally the concentration of calcium in cells is regulated by the actions of calcium-binding proteins (CaBPs), which latch on to excess calcium ions. There is no question calcium-binding proteins are important for regulating the calcium concentrations within the cells. The key factor is the cell's "neurons." Neurons are specialized cells, not just in humans but also in animals that, as units of the nervous system, carry information by receiving and transmitting electrical impulses. Studies have also shown neurons that lack certain calcium-binding proteins are less able to handle chemical stressors to their systems - such as too much calcium.

And how can cells get too much calcium? A decrease in the number of calcium-binding proteins in our bodies can result in too much calcium within our cells, which accelerates the aging process, chronic or acute inflammation, and the onset of serious neurological diseases.

With such an important role in the functioning of the brain, it's not surprising that calcium has been intensely studied in the fields of learning, memory, and aging. Over the last fifteen years, scientists are starting to believe that a breakdown in regulating calcium is a major factor in the development of aging-related learning and memory problems seen in many species, including humans. Research has also shown that calcium-dependent processes are important for associative learning in both adult and aged animals. Other scientists indicate that using compounds that block the influx of calcium, such as calcium channel blockers, actually improves learning and memory. Administering medication to control the rates of calcium entry into neurons has also been proven somewhat helpful in boosting the cognitive thinking of older people.

Many other studies suggest a selective decrease in certain calcium-binding proteins occurs in the brains of aged animals, including humans. Loss of these important proteins with advancing age may leave neurons vulnerable to even moderate increases in the amount of intracellular calcium. The relationship between calcium, neuron degeneration, calcium-binding proteins, and aging suggests that replenishing these proteins in the neurons, through supplementation, especially in parts of the brain that are known to degenerate with advancing age such as the hippocampus, will slow the effects of aging.

Through its use in scientific laboratories around the world, Aequorin has proved to be completely safe and has never shown any dangerous effects.

Because Aequorin binds to calcium inside cells, it is classified as a calcium-binding protein. Many other calcium-binding proteins exist in all the cells in our body and thus have the ability to regulate and control biological processes that involve calcium.

What conclusions can we reach, as the result of all these scientific studies – all of which have shown the same positive results? Let's reprise our findings, step by step:

Step one: In neurodegenerative diseases -- that is, problems within the body stemming from trouble within the neurons -- there is a known depletion in neuroprotective calcium-binding proteins, which correlates directly with the progression and increasing severity of the disease.

Step two: This strongly suggests that calcium-binding proteins serve an important role in protecting neurons from calcium overload and keeping the cellular circuitry firing properly.

Step three: The easiest way to replenish the calcium-binding proteins that we lose as we age, or fight disease, is with Aequorin. (If that word is still a tough one to remember, think of the commercial product Prevagen or another that has an Aequorin base.

The technology used to produce Aequorin supplements is now commonplace in the manufacturing of many nutraceuticals and over-the-counter dietary supplements. Testing is ongoing and seems to be universally favorable. In a recent test, single doses given orally to laboratory rats produced absolutely no toxic or adverse symptoms. All test animals were thoroughly examined for any changes in the tissue pathology or cells of various internal organs, and absolutely no adverse reactions were found.

In short: Aequorin has been used in laboratory studies for more than three decades with no adverse reactions, but only until recently could enough be manufactured to demonstrate these higher levels of safety. Scientists using Aequorin to measure calcium levels inside cells have long known that it produces no ill effects in experimental animals, and no damage to any cells exposed to Aequorin has ever been reported.

So anyone facing the problem of aging – and that's everyone – should be aware of this neurological heavyweight, the champion battling enemies such as Alzheimer's and Parkinson's on our behalf. That is the easy, safe, and economical way to replenish the calcium-binding proteins that your own body produces, and then loses, as all of us age.

CHAPTER TWO

Andrographis paniculata

Andrographis paniculata:
The MASTER immune booster

Andrographis Paniculata (AP)? What does this mean? It certainly doesn't conjure up any images for you or me. But just to give you something in English: Andrographis Paniculata is commonly known as "The King of Bitters." Why? For its bitter taste. Don't let this bother you though, it's the one nutrient you'll want in your medicine cabinet at all times.

That's right. Throw out the aspirin, pain meds, anti-inflammatories, "tums," laxatives, anti-diarrheas, sedatives, cough medicines, and antibacterial creams because you won't need them anymore. This natural nutrient is rated #1 in medicinal properties.

Not only won't you find any better natural ingredient for the immediate relief for the ailments I just mentioned - but Andrographis Paniculata (AP) shields and helps rid your body of some very serious diseases.

These benefits include:

- Counteracting intermittent diseases such as Malaria
- Inhibiting viral activity
- Protecting your heart muscles
- Purifying and cleansing your blood
- Promoting easy digestion
- Reducing blood sugar levels
- Protecting the liver and gallbladder
- Increasing white cell phagocytosis
- Inhibiting HIV-1 replication and increasing T cell and T lymphocyte counts
- Killing intestinal worms
- Fighting and even killing cancer cells
- Treating herpes
- Treating Alzheimer's disease
- Contributing to healthy joints
- Counteracting the effects of rheumatoid arthritis

Andrographis Paniculata - aka "The King of Bitters" was extensively researched in the 80's and 90's confirming its outstanding and extremely beneficial properties. Before Western medicine acquainted itself with AP's medicinal benefits, Chinese Medicine had already incorporated its uses, and AP had already been used for centuries in 26 Ayurvedic formulas for not one but as you can see, several medical traditions.

The Plant

A member of the Acantaceae, AP is an annual growing anywhere from
½ to 1 meter in height. Its leaves and stems are used to extract its active
phytochemicals. Grown from seeds, AP is indigenous in India, Pakistan and
Indonesia. You can find it growing wild in evergreen and forest areas, even
along the roadsides.

Its primary medicinal component is Andrographolide, its leaves containing the
highest amount. But does it really work? Or is it merely folk medicine?

AP the immune booster and battler of cancer

AP is a highly potent immune stimulator for two reasons:

1. AP initiates an antigen-specific response. (Meaning it generates antibodies, which our bodies need in order to counteract invading microbes.)
2. AP initiates a non-specific immune response. (Macrophage cells scavenge
   and destroy harmful invaders.)

What does this mean to you and me? In simple terms, Antigens originate within
the body or from the outside environment. The immune system provides two
lines of defense: nonspecific and specific immune responses.

A first-time encounter with an antigen elicits a nonspecific immune response.
Defense mechanisms include skin, mucous membranes, chemicals, specialized
cells, and the inflammatory response. Unbroken skin is a formidable physical
barrier to most antigens.

Mucous membranes line body cavities such as the mouth and stomach. These
structures secrete saliva and hydrochloric acid, respectively, chemicals that
destroy bacteria. If antigens pass through the defenses, a variety of white blood
cells such as macrophages, neutrophils, and mast cells try to destroy them. Other
mechanisms in the blood such as antibacterial proteins, interferon (antiviral
proteins), and natural killer cells aid in the battle.

A specific immune response is elicited when an antigen invades the body that it
has previously encountered.

The andrographolides are found to enhance the immune system by:
• Producing white blood cells "the pac man" of bacteria and foreign matter.
• Releasing interferon (a protein called cytokine made by cells to fight viruses).
• Influencing activity of the lymph system.

AP the natural cancer-fighting agent

When cancer upsets normal development, our cells don't mature and more closely resemble immature body cells. The more they resemble immature cells, the more unfavorable the outcome: the cancer grows and spread more rapidly.

AP extracts derived from the components of its leaves (andrographolides) can kill cancer cells. This "cancer cell-killer" is clearly demonstrated against human epidermal carcinoma of the skin lining and against lymphocytic leukemia cells. AP's ability to kill cancer cells was found to be superior to the levels of effectiveness recommended by the National Cancer Institute.

A Japanese research study reported AP stopped stomach cancer cells from multiplying. After three days of the study, there were less than 8 cancer cells growing with the presence of AP, while the untreated cancer cells numbered 120.

Another group of Japanese researchers tested AP on sarcoma cells. These very malignant cancers affect muscle, connective, tissue, and bones. When tumor samples were examined under the microscope, AP was found to inhibit the growth of these types of tumors.

Better yet: These AP extracts are much less toxic than most chemotherapeutic agents used to fight cancer.

AP's anti-viral benefits on HIV and other viruses

HIV, like all viruses can't reproduce themselves, or even live, without using the cell's resources. When the HIV virus finds a suitable cell it attaches to the cell by way of proteins on its cell surface. The HIV virus sneaks its way into the cells by binding two molecules on the cell's surface.

How HIV works: HIV tends to be drawn to the brain and certain skin tissues. It also forms an attack on the immune system and debilitates the cells. Helper T cells are the main target of the virus, (T representing the Thymus gland where the cells are produced). These cells signal the lymph nodes and the spleen to produce more antibodies against the HIV virus. Once the antibodies inactivate the virus, suppressor T cells produce chemicals that stop further production of antibodies. But the HIV virus, attaches itself to the helper T cell. There the virus tricks the T cell into producing chemicals the virus feeds on. HIV then takes over the "brain" of the T cell and turns into a virus production factory that's no longer part of the immune system. Without T cells, other components of our immune system don't receive messages to produce more antibodies and our resistance is compromised.

Research: Cooperative research at the National Cancer Institute showed that andrographolides could inhibit HIV's toxic effect on cells by inhibiting c-mos, (a genetic component involved in HIV growth and T-cell death). C-mos integrates itself into the DNA of a cell and usually is inactive.

Normally found only in reproductive system cells, c-mos isn't expressed in CD4 (protein markers on the surface of certain types of T lymphocytes) or other body cells. For this to happen, an enzyme (c-mos kinase) is needed. Andrographis extract can inhibit this enzyme so that it can help support normal immune function. It's thought that the action of AP in AIDS is that the herbal extract appears to induce programmed cancer cell death. This process helps the cells to break up into particles, which are then scavenged by immune system cells.

The tests done at the Frederick Research Center demonstrate that AP extracts increased AZT's (an antiviral that slows HIV infection) ability to inhibit replication of HIV. The AP and AZT combination was greater than that of either compound used alone. An added benefit to this is that lower doses of AZT can be used.

Throw out the cold medicine.
It's true. AP used in a double-blind study showed AP to be a strong preventive measure against the common cold. A group of students were given "Kan Jang" (a formulation of AP produced by the Swedish Herbal Institute). The students were diagnosed for the presence or absence of colds during a three-month period. A dose of 200mg a day was given to the study group. After one month there was no significant difference in the number of colds. But - after the third month of taking AP there was a significant decrease in the incidence of colds as compared to a placebo group. The students who received the AP formulation had a 30% rate incidence of colds compared to 62% of students receiving the placebo. The preventive effect could be due to the presence of andrographolide, with its known immuno-stimulant effects.

Existing colds. The amount of AP formulation used in the previous study was much less than was used in this cited study that produced quicker results. In this study, patients were divided into two groups: One was given 1,200mg a day (these patients already had colds, including runny noses, nasal congestion, sore throats, muscle aches, earaches, cough, fevers, and headaches). The other group was given a placebo. The beginning of the study showed that those taking AP and those taking the placebo showed similar symptoms. But after the fourth day researchers found that AP accelerated the recuperation of these patients.

Throw out the aspirin and anti-inflammatories
Fever, pain reduction, and inflammation - no problem.

AP's innate ability as a fever reducer has been demonstrated time and again in several laboratories. Studies done in China have shown that andrographolide, neondrgraholide, and dehydroandrographolide can lower fever produced by many different fever-inducing agents.

Safer than aspirin. AP extracts produce the same results of 200mg of aspirin/kg body weight. Also established was that there was a wider margin of safety using AP extracts which is a good indication of its lack of toxicity.

Inflammation caused by histamine, dimethyl benzene, hemolytic necrosis, and acute pneumocystis produced by adrenaline was significantly reduced or relieved with AP. The effect was found in all major andrographolides: andrographolide, neoandrographolide, and dehydroandrographolide. Dehydroandrographolide had the most profound effect followed by the other two AP components. The anti-inflammatory action was due to its effect that AP had on increasing the synthesis and release of andrenocorticotrophic (ACTH) hormone of the pituitary gland of the brain. ACTH signals the adrenal gland to make cortisol, a natural anti-inflammatory. AP was found to inhibit edema as well.

Throw out the antibiotics
The anti-bacterial uses of AP are especially important today because of bacteria becoming resistant to the drugs we have on the market. Each time bacteria are exposed to an antibiotic, most are killed, but a few survive. These survivors multiply and create infections that can't be treated with the typical antibiotic, and in some cases no existing drugs stop can stop the bacteria. AP and other herbs complement the effects of antibiotics. Natural remedies combined with synthetic medication used in therapies are more effective and safer.

Throw out the Imodium
Diarrhea-type diseases are one of the top ten causes of death worldwide and the leading cause of death in children of developing countries. The drugs used to relieve the symptoms of diarrhea (i.e., kaolin-pectin, Lomotil, Imodium and others), have extremely undesirable side effects. AP extracts significantly effect diarrhea associated with E. coli bacterial infections. AP components show a similar activity to Imodium the most common anti-diarrheal drug.

Aid for Cardiovascular disease:
AP keeps blood and oxygen flowing to the brain

Clot dissolving drugs used in emergency treatment of heart attacks appear to be as effective as angioplasty and may prevent heart attacks or strokes occurring with one month of angioplasty. Research conducted to better understand the signals involved in bleeding and blood vessel development is making use of signal transduction technology (described later in this chapter). Rather than drugs, AP shows significant promise in preventing blood vessels from constricting.

Another way to prevent cardiovascular disease is to correct high blood pressure. Researchers have reported that an extract of AP produces an anti-hypertension effect by relaxing the smooth muscles in the walls of the blood vessels. This relaxation effect prevents the blood vessels from constricting and limiting blood flow to the heart, brain, and other organs in the body. AP keeps the blood and oxygen flowing to the brain. The symptoms of diminished blood flow to the brain are short-term memory loss, ringing in the ears, dizziness, headaches, depression and impaired mental performance. Another benefit is that AP's effects aren't toxic. It's inexpensive as well, which combined, makes AP treatment the miracle herb for cardiovascular therapy.

AP protects the liver and gallbladder

Liver: Twenty-six different formulas in Ayurvedic medicine contain AP compounds for liver disorders. AP's four related medicinal compounds were tested to find out whether or not they could fight against liver toxicity. During testing, mice were given a cleaning solvent, alcohol, or other toxic chemicals. The free radicals produced by these chemical attacks on the body destroyed cellular membranes that surround liver cells. When the AP compounds were given to animals three days before the toxic chemicals were ingested, there was a huge protective effect on the liver. The effect was attributed to the antioxidant ability of the AP compounds.

Infectious hepatitis is an acute inflammatory condition of the liver. It's often followed by liver cirrhosis and may progress to coma and death. In India, a group of physicians used AP to treat similar liver ailments. When the study was conducted to evaluate the effect of AP, it showed a marked improvement in the majority of patients given an infusion of AP.

Gallbladder: AP stimulates gallbladder function. In animal experiments, those that received andrographolides for seven consecutive days showed an increase in bile flow, bile salts, and bile acids -- extremely beneficial for enhanced gallbladder function - showing that AP may decrease the probability of gallstone formation and might also aid fat digestion.

Nervous System disorders

Not many compounds penetrate the blood-brain barrier. AP does. It concentrates in the blood and especially in the spinal cord. Several studies show us that AP has a sedative effect. Mice given barbital as an anesthetic became sedated more quickly and it lasted longer. But given with AP, it became possible to give the mice less anesthesia when it was given along with AP. Concluding that AP may act on the barbital receptors in the brain.

AP and its respiratory effects

AP is sometimes used to treat tonsillitis, respiratory infections, and tuberculosis. Examples: AP used to treat 129 cases of tonsillitis: 65% of the patients responded to the therapy. Using AP to treat 49 pneumonia patients: 40 cases showed positive changes and 9 patients completely recovered. Another example: One hundred eleven patients with pneumonia, and 20 with chronic bronchitis and lung infection were given AP – the overall effectiveness of the AP treatment was 91%.

Proof Positive

AP's extensive research is centered on what's called "signal transduction technology" which shows us how AP works with the cells within the body – especially throughout the viscera.

Here's a good explanation of first - what signal transduction is. I'll quote Jean Barilla, MS: "All cells in our body contain receptors on the surface of the cell membrane that surrounds the cell. These receptors work to bind hormones, growth factors, neurotransmitters, and other molecules to regulate (or in the case of cancer, disturb) cell function.

Once a molecule binds to the receptor, they transmit a chemical message to the targets in the cell or other molecules in the cell, which carry the message even further. Its message eventually reaches the nucleus of the cell where the genetic material (DNA) is stored. The DNA is activated and the cell responds according to what type of cell it is. An example would be a message transmitted to make a particular protein, such as insulin, by a cell in the pancreas. The receptor, its cellular target, and any intermediary molecules are referred to as Signal Transduction."

Today, we can find out what can go wrong at this very basic level inside the cells, so researchers have a better chance to detect disease at a much earlier stage. This affords us the chance to correct the problem before it gets out of hand. Here's how the process works:

Signal Transduction Technology

Life scientists have long sought to understand how signals make their way through the body's pathways. In recent years their search has taken on added urgency as it has become clear that signal transduction holds the key in treating human disease. "Pathogenic organisms have learned to use these signaling pathways in human cells to their advantage," explains Tony Pawson, Co-Director of the Samuel Lunenfeld Research Institute at Toronto's Mount Sinai Hospital. "As we understand more about signaling we can learn how to reverse the damage. If we can lay out the wiring diagram of human cells in a comprehensive way, we can play engineer and repair the cells when things go wrong."

Signal transduction technology helps determine the effects of natural and synthetic components on the signal transduction pathways in the cell, particularly those involved in cell division. Applications of signal transduction technology are used to develop compounds for therapeutic potential.

Naturally, the criticisms made by conventional medical and scientific communities to refute natural supplements are that they're based on folklore, not science. But by using signal transduction technology to investigate the effect on botanicals or other nutritional supplements on the cellular level is good science and irrefutable.

This level of investigation certainly legitimizes the nutritional approach in prevention and treatment of disease and speeds up the process of development of new and more effective supplements.

Using the signal transduction technology on AP extracts, shows AP counteracts the interferences in the cell cycle. Interferences in the cell cycle are the basis for developing cancer or infection with such viruses as HIV-1.

We can draw this conclusion:

Because of AP's wide distribution in our tissues and organ distribution and the immune-stimulating and regulatory actions, AP is an ideal candidate in preventing and treating many diseases and conditions. The biological effects and potential treatment properties previously discussed makes Andrographis a master immune system enhancer.

My personal recommendation:

ParActin® made by Herbal Power. It's the only supplement that holds the patent in the cultivation and manufacture of the true Andrographis Paniculata.

CHAPTER THREE

Carnosine

Carosine
A Gift from Nature: The Fountain of Youth

If you've never heard of Carnosine before now, I know you'll want to add it to your vocabulary and your daily routine. If you have already heard of Carnosine, you already use it … because you know it's the most potent age-defying, antioxidant ever discovered.

The anti-aging benefits of Carnosine are touted around the world for its genuine "fountain of youth" properties.

What's even more astounding is this: "Mother Nature" provides every living organism, creature, and plant with the capability to produce Carnosine in his, her or its body. Yes, the joke is on us! Those legends in search of the "fountain of youth" rarely intimate that it can be found inside the universe of our very own bodies.

What is Carnosine?

Carnosine is a 100% natural multi-use antioxidant. It's a very simple, yet powerful dipeptide (a molecule consisting of two amino acids joined together by a single peptide bond). The specific amino acids that make up Carnosine are beta-alanine and histidine. All of your cells -- especially the cells in your muscles, heart, brain and connective tissue – produce Carnosine.

> **Noteworthy caveat:**
> Carnosine levels in your body decline by 63% between the ages of 10 and70 years old. It seems that people who live longer tend to produce and retain more Carnosine in their cells than those with a shorter lifespan. This may point the finger at the main cause of age-related deterioration in muscle mass as well.

The not-so-good news: Carnosine levels decline quickly, starting at age 10 and sliding downhill between the ages of 10 and 70.

The really good news: We can supplement the decline of Carnosine and bring the levels back up.

Carnosine's restorative benefits include:

- A more youthful appearance.
- Increasing mental acuity.
- Increasing endurance and strength levels.
- Regulating hormone levels.
- Preventing muscle fatigue.
- Improving muscle mass in the elderly.
- Lowering blood pressure.
- Protecting cataract formation.
- Reducing and preventing cell damage from beta amyloid in Alzheimer patients.
- Improving the immune system and healing wounds.
- Killing organisms that cause ulcers and stomach cancer.
- Improving social skills and speech in children with autism.
- Warding off tumors.

> **Noteworthy:**
> *Carnosine is the only antioxidant to significantly protect chromosomes from oxidative damages due to 90% oxygen exposure.*

Carnosine's uncanny ability to make old cells YOUNG again:

Carnosine actually reverses the signs of aging in your cells. Its newly-discovered capacity to take old cells and make them young again gives it the power to not only make you look younger and prolong your life span, but give you the energy to make your life more vital as well. It's as close to a miraculous supplement as you can find. And yes, it's readily available.

What makes us look older?

1. Oxidation.
2. AGE (Advanced Glycosylation End Products).
3. Chronic inflammation.
4. Hormonal deregulation.

> *Experts say: Carnosine should be made a daily treatment for people of all ages, especially those over 40 years old.*

When our bodies begin showing signs of age, it's a fair bet that proteins (which make up a major part of our body) have already started altering and literally turning against our bodies. Once these proteins start altering themselves through oxidation and interactions with sugar (aldehydes) – they change at an alarming rate. Now the proteins actually become destructive. And as we age, about a third of the proteins in our bodies become altered. These protein modifications include oxidation, carbonylation (an accumulation of proteins with carbonyl groups), cross-linking, glycation (when glucose and proteins link and bind together), and Advanced Glycation End Product (AGE) formation (which accelerates the aging process and quite possibly promote degenerative diseases). Karin Granstrom Jordan, M.D.'s description of AGE in her article: Carnosine: Nature's pluripotent life extension agent is one of the best descriptions of "AGE":

"AGE formation in the body is the chemical equivalent of the browning of food in the oven – and equally irreversible…," Carnosine keeps AGE formation in the body from building, and also protects normal proteins from the toxic effects of AGEs that have already formed."

Carnosine's Reprieve: The road to rejuvenation

In the past we could only stand by and witness the accumulation of typical signs of aging and disease: Wrinkled skin, degeneration of our eyes, as well as neuro-degeneration. These damaged proteins accumulate and cross-link in the skin, causing wrinkles and the loss of elasticity. (Cross-linking proteins are a major cause of cataracts as well.)

Today we have a reprieve: Carnosine holds the innate power to gobble up and flush out free radical groups … such as singlet oxygen, hydrogen peroxide, peroxyl, and hydroxyl radicals, and an over-abundance of zinc and copper metals, from causing more damage.

Carnosine also protects against formation of warped cellular proteins that have been damaged by sugar (aldehydes), and from carbonylation and other protein modifications we discussed earlier.

Not only is Carnosine known for its ability to flush out toxins, but it seems to react to the modified proteins in ways that some researchers suggest may make the proteins easier to break up and disposed of by the cell's "garbage disposal" system. Carnosine also helps maintain the integrity and complex internal structure of our cells.

Simple antioxidants (E and C) are out of their league when they try to combat the complexities of protein modifications. Carnosine is, however, in a league of its own and is proven to be the safeguard against these protein modifications.

Carnosine: the gate-keeper of our youth

Drs. Gail McFarland and Robin Holliday from the Australia Commonwealth Scientific and Industrial Research

> *Carnosine reduces and prevents cell damage and actually makes older cells amazingly young again.*

Organization embarked on a simple experiment and made a discovery that literally has rocked the world of science:

The experiment:

Drs. McFarland and Holliday took human fibroblasts (connective tissue cells) from the lung and foreskin and placed half the cells into a standard cell culture environment without Carnosine; they then took the remaining half and placed them into the same type of standard cell culture with Carnosine.

The discovery:

The Carnosine-supplemented fibroblasts reproduced themselves much longer (up to one to seven more population-doublings). Plus, the cells lived longer (up to two thirds longer) than the cells in the standard environment without Carnosine.

There was something else the medical team found, too. The Carnosine-supplemented cell culture made the cells YOUNGER than they had been.

Yes, it's authenticated.

McFarland and Holliday stated: "...Striking effects on the cell's shape and structure. Carnosine preserved the cells' youthful shapes. The cells raised in the usual medium (standard culture without Carnosine) got old, blotchy, and irregular and broke apart into scattered islands of twisted debris.

"Yet the fibroblasts raised in Carnosine still have the same appearance they had when they were young: the colonies are flat, with their youthful whorling patterns; they're smooth, regular, and even. Remarkably, cells bathed in Carnosine stayed youthful almost until the very end of their lives."

Turning back time

Does Carnosine really reverse the signs of aging and make cells YOUNGER?

McFarland and Holliday took the fibroblasts from the Carnosine medium and moved them into the standard non-Carnosine culture. Naturally, they grew old. And here's the fascinating part – when they placed these same fibroblasts back into the Carnosine bath, they sprang back to life.

Here's how the doctors explained it: "Switching the fibroblasts between media with and without Carnosine also switches their phenotype (visibly observable properties) from aged to juvenile, and the reverse ... proposing that Carnosine is an important component of cellular maintenance mechanisms."

> *Surprising anti-cancerous effects found in Carnosine: While MacFarland was working on cell-rejuvenation she stumbled onto something that completely surprised everyone. She noticed one of the cell cultures had become infected with cancer cells, quickly choking out the healthy cells. When she added Carnosine to the samples, the cell cultures returned to normal health. She then tested Carnosine against seven human cancer cell lines and found that after adding cancerous cells to a culture of healthy cells bathed in Carnosine, the cancer cells slowly disappeared from the pool, even while the healthy cells thrived.*

This points to Carnosine as a heavy player in keeping cells in the tightly-regulated condition, helping them function at optimal capacity.

Will Carnosine make you look younger and live longer?

Here's an interesting study: In a recent study in Russia, MO Yuneva and colleagues gave a group of SAM mice Carnosine-supplemented drinking water, beginning at two months of age (adjusting for metabolic consideration, about one gram per day). The second group of SAM mice was given just regular water.

What happened next is great news for you and me:
The mice with the Carnosine-supplemented drinking water lived 20% longer, on average, than the non-Carnosine-supplemented mice. The maximum survival rate was 6% longer.

In simple terms: that's adding five years to your life.

The mice looked and acted younger throughout their lives compared to those without the Carnosine supplement.
Here's what the studies showed when they compared the Carnosine supplemented group with those that were given no Carnosine:

- More than 40% kept the color and vitality of their hair.
- 61% showed no signs of skin ulcers.
- A decrease in senile spinal curvature occurred by 13%.
- They had significantly less or lack of lesions around the eyes, as is common when we age.

- The mice performed 29% better on tests for passive avoidance.
- Mice performed 6½ times better on tests that measured youthful exploratory curiosity.

The positive conclusion: In a recent professional article, Dr. Marios Kyriazis found that his patients who were taking Carnosine supplements enjoyed comments that they simply look younger. This may be a reflection of the phenomenon observed in these SAM mice. Carnosine supplements made these mice much more resistant to the features of aging. They lived longer and retained their youthful appearance, and maintained physiological good health and normal behavior, as well as extended the life span in SAM mice.

Carnosine helps defend the brain from losing its mind

Nature planted a considerable amount of Carnosine in our brains just to protect them from cell damage and brain degeneration. It also works as a neurotransmitter, anti-convulsant, and flushing device for toxic metals. It's a versatile neuroprotectant against all neurological and psychiatric syndromes and disorders as well.

Carnosine plays a huge role in modulating brain cell function by simultaneously making neurons more sensitive to certain signals and protecting neuron toxicity from over-stimulation.

Here's a perfect example:

When Russian biochemist M.O. Yuneva and fellow researchers measured the indicators associated with brain aging in the SAM mice, they found that the brain membranes of the Carnosine-treated mice had significantly less MDA (malonidialdehyde), a highly toxic product of lipid oxidation than those mice given water without the Carnosine. They also found that Carnosine therapy increased the binding of the brain messenger glutamate (the main excitatory neurotransmitter) to the N-methyl-D-aspartate receptor (NMDA), (crucial for long-term memory).

This is good news, because if glutamate (the main excitatory neurotransmitter) is not bound with NMDA, excessive glutamate can become toxic, creating excitotoxicity, which can cause membrane polarization, ending in cell death.

The importance of this discovery is this: Carnosine helped in binding glutamate to its NMDA receptors and may explain the normal behavioral reactivity in the SAM mice. Remember, only 9% of the untreated mice displayed normal behavioral reactivity, compared to 58% of the Carnosine treated mice. We can conclude that Carnosine offers protection against the damaging effects of excitotoxicity.

> "In Alzheimer's disease, lipid peroxidation products are thought to interfere with critical membrane proteins involved in cellular signaling and in transporting ions, glucose and glutamate. Their impairment leads to membrane depolarization, metabolic deficit, excitotoxicity and increased vulnerability to oxidative assault." (Mark RJ et al)

The trade secret of the athletes

It's a little frightening to think about what happens to our body mass, strength and endurance between the ages of 20-70 years. Our body structure starts declining by 20%! The concentration and antioxidant effect in our bodies decreases by half as we increase in age.

There's an enemy in our camp … leaving its mark by reducing muscle mass, strength, and endurance. Weak and atrophied muscle fibers have been found to include very little Carnosine. The Australian team, led by MacFarland, recently showed that supplementation with Carnosine increases the strength and endurance of tired muscles. Carnosine plays a central role in keeping muscle cells contracting and preventing fatigue, fending off lactic acid, and allowing isolated muscle cells that have been pushed beyond their workload limits to contract again. The more Carnosine you take, the higher the content in your muscles.

That's why Carnosine is the ideal supplement among athletes:

- Carnosine inhibits lactic acid build-up,
- Carnosine helps detoxify the muscles during physical endurance,
- Carnosine protects the muscles from injury,
- Carnosine increases muscle strength and endurance,
- Carnosine speeds up the recovery process after strenuous exercise.

Athletes or not – our bodies could all benefit from a lot of that.

The eyes have it:

The benefits of Carnosine for the eyes are remarkable. Here's how. Carnosine:

- Reduces, reverses, and slows down the occurrence of senile cataracts.
- Lowers intraocular pressure associated with glaucoma.
- Helps those with contact lens disorders.
- Combats eyestrain.
- Alleviates symptoms of presbyopia (progressive form of farsightedness that affects most people by the age of 60 or earlier.
- Eases computer vision syndrome.
- Ends discomfort of ocular inflammation.
- Restores normal sight for those inflicted with blurred vision.
- Alleviates dry eye syndrome.
- Fights against retinal diseases.
- Treats vitreous opacities and lesions.

Did you know that 5.5 million people have eyesight interference? The culprit: Cataracts. And 400,000 are newly diagnosed with them every year.

I used to tell my patients: Once you get cataracts there isn't much you can do about it…Today, thanks to research centering on Carnosine, you have the chance to improve cataracts and the overall health of your eyes.

How much Carnosine should I take?

I'm a Carnosine user myself. I take between 2-4,000mg per day for anti-aging purposes. And yes, I can feel the difference.

Studies also show that feeding animals Carnosine in dosages equivalent to a human taking over four hundred milligrams of Carnosine a day had no effect on the Carnosine levels in muscles, heart, or the liver; while higher dosages increase Carnosine levels in muscles and have clear therapeutic benefits to the brain and the body. You should understand that the exact cutoff point is uncertain, and indeed may vary from one individual to another. Benefits clearly and consistently emerge at dosages equivalent to about 1,000 milligrams per day and up, for a person of average height.

You can supplement Carnosine in food sources such as, meat, poultry, and fish (though there are fewer and fewer of us eating meat today). In recent years we've seen a massive decline in the amount of meat we eat, not to mention the deterioration of the "quality" of our meat sources, so it stands to reason: less Carnosine is found in our diets today.

Now, do I need to ask?

By supplementing our diets with Carnosine we get a huge reprieve. Its life-prolonging agent slows down the aging processes. And in a society where Alzheimer's disease is increasing, more people having strokes, and an alarming number of people are being diagnosed with cancer, we need to ensure that our body gets the nutrients it needs to prevent these diseases.

CHAPTER FOUR

Cell Oxygenation

Cellular Nutrition = Oxygen, Hydrogen, Minerals

Besides breathing, why do we need oxygen?

All functions of our body are regulated by oxygen. Oxygen energizes cells so they can regenerate. Our body uses oxygen to metabolize food and to eliminate toxins and waste through oxidation. Our brain needs oxygen every second to process information. The ability to think, feel, move, eat, sleep and even talk depends on energy generated from oxygen.

Oxygen is the only element capable of combining with almost every other element to form the essential components necessary to build and maintain our bodies. For instance, oxygen + nitrogen + carbon + hydrogen = proteins. Oxygen + carbon + hydrogen = carbohydrates. Oxygen + hydrogen = water. The combination of oxygen in the air, water, proteins and carbohydrates creates life energy. None of this energy could be produced without oxygen.

Life's breath

Life is propelled by the oxygen in our blood— and a lack of oxygen results in sickness, poor vitality, poor stamina, fatigue and a general weak disposition.

Our normal level of oxygen reserves can be depleted by a number of factors including:

- **Toxic Stress** - toxic chemicals and air pollution, both becoming more prevalent in our industrialized cities, and increased use of antibiotics;
- **Emotional Stress** - produces adrenaline and adrenal-related hormones, which utilize more oxygen;
- **Physical Trauma** - reduces circulation and oxygen supply to many cells and tissues throughout the body;
- **Infections** - use up "free radical" forms of oxygen to fight bacteria, fungi and viruses. Frequent use of drugs also depletes our oxygen supplies at the cellular level.

Noted authorities stress that most diseases, especially yeast or fungal infections, occur most frequently in any oxygen-poor environment in the body.

(Warning: Atmospheric oxygen concentration levels are being reduced by nearly one percent every 15 years or so.)

Are you oxygen deficient?
Oxygen therapy can overcome that deficiency

Initial symptoms of oxygen deficiency may include overall weakness, fatigue, circulation problems, poor digestion, muscle aches, dizziness, depression, memory loss, irrational behavior, irritability, acid stomach, and bronchial complications. When the immune system is compromised by a lack of oxygen, the body is more susceptible to opportunistic bacteria, viral, and parasitic infections, colds, and flu. Oxygen deprivation can trigger life-threatening diseases— as underscored by a medical authority's assertion that cancer and other infections or diseases cannot live in an oxygen-rich environment.

Oxygen acts as a guardian and protector against unfriendly bacteria and disease organisms that invade your body. Rubble, garbage, toxins, refuse, debris, and any useless substances are destroyed by oxygen and carried out of the system. When not enough oxygen is present, consider "oxygen therapy."

Oxygen therapy is any supplemental process that safely increases the available dissolved oxygen content in the body. Some of the accepted oxygen therapies:

- **Bottled Oxygen** is often prescribed as inhalation therapy for serious bronchial and other respiratory problems.

- **Ozone (O3) Therapy** generally infused rectally or intravenously is primarily used to increase blood oxygenation, circulation, immunity, and to kill bacteria, viruses and fungi. Warning: Ozone oxygen is extremely unstable and can be toxic if not administered properly.

- **Hydrogen Peroxide (H2O2) Therapy** - Hydrogen peroxide is manufactured in the bloodstream to help fight bacteria, viruses, yeast, fungi, and other invading pathogens. The ingestion of H2O2 is controversial because it can cause an adverse reaction in the digestive tract. This therapy should be utilized only under the supervision of a licensed health care professional.

- **Hyperbaric Oxygen Therapy** involves breathing oxygen in a pressurized chamber. This therapy saturates tissues and cells with oxygen, thereby greatly enhancing healing and immune-system response. HBO therapy was originally designed to treat divers and aviators for decompression sickness and air embolisms. Today HBO therapy is helpful in treating a wide variety of diseases, pathogens and degenerative conditions.

Many oxygen products tend to flood the body with oxygen, often creating harmful oxygen free radicals. So an opinion: The easiest and most cost effective form of oxygen therapy is the daily ingestion of CellFood Dietary Supplement. It's the one form that does not create free radicals - in fact, it actually uses them to create more stable oxygen. More about that ahead.

The Master Builder: Hydrogen

Hydrogen is the most abundant element in the universe. It is estimated to make up more than 90% of all the atoms - three quarters of the mass of the universe!

Hydrogen is the simplest element known to man. Each atom of hydrogen has only one proton. It is also the most plentiful gas in the universe. Stars are made primarily of hydrogen.

The sun is basically a giant ball of hydrogen and helium gases. In the sun's core, hydrogen atoms combine to form helium atoms. This process - called fusion - gives off radiant energy. This radiant energy sustains life on earth. It gives us light and makes plants grow. It makes the wind blow and rain fall. It is stored as chemical energy in fossil fuels. Most of the energy we use today came from the sun's radiant energy.

Most body processes require hydrogen. Hydrogen builds cells … but if left unmodulated, makes them hard and brittle. These effects are balanced by the action of oxygen.

The body normally obtains hydrogen from water, other liquids, fruits, and vegetables. A lack of hydrogen can lead to dehydration - causing extreme dryness and abnormal nerve heat generation inside the body. Because of dehydration, moisture and fatty nutrients are not well assimilated; this may result in brain shrinkage, face furrowing, drying of mucus, and tendon/nerve cramping. Other conditions caused by a lack of hydrogen include gout, muscular rheumatism, mental confusion and inadequacy, neck stiffness, irritated skin, and sore joints.

The Ocean of Life: Water

Ah, H2O. Everybody knows that means water. Everybody knows the "H" is for hydrogen and the "O" is for oxygen.

Scientists estimate that humans can live no more than three days without water— such is the importance of this element. All chemical reactions in the body take place in water. Every cell in the body is bathed in water, which contains materials to keep them vibrant. Water is the transporter of nutrients and oxygen for proper function of the body's tissues; it helps remove waste from the body; it acts as a natural air conditioner through perspiration; it's essential for digestion and absorption of vitamins and minerals. Water keeps our skin moist and supple and is a natural lubricator for our joints and internal organs.

Over the course of an average day, the body loses approximately three quarts of water through breathing, perspiration, and elimination. Through strenuous exercise or on a hot day, however, our bodies can lose as much as three quarts of water each hour. This fluid must be replaced or muscle cramping, dehydration, or heat stroke may take place. Water is involved in every bodily function, so it's hardly surprising that dehydration can lead to mental and physical breakdown.

The growing pollution in our modern day world is having an increasingly detrimental effect on our drinking water. Hazardous chemicals like mercury, lead, arsenic, cyanide, aluminum and phosphorus are getting into the water system every day. Other dangerous and toxic chemicals, including chlorine and fluoride, are added to reduce harmful microorganisms and prevent tooth problems. All this adds to the load of toxins that our bodies have to eliminate.

For cleansing and nourishing our cells, we need half our body's weight in fluid ounces per day (and more if we want to lose weight). This doesn't include coffee, tea, alcohol, fruit juice, or other liquids. Dehydration causes bodily functions to go into distress because fewer toxins are being removed, and less oxygen and nutrients can be transported throughout the body— especially to the brain, which is about 75% water.

For good quality drinking water, we need to purify or filter the water before drinking it. Boiling water is not effective because although it kills the pathogens, it concentrates the pollutants that are in the water. Start with the best quality water available to get the greatest benefits possible.

The Riches of the Earth: Minerals

We need, in proper quantities and proportions, more than 70 minerals for peak performance of every cell in our body – for the proper composition of the body fluids, for the formation of blood and bone cells, and for healthy nerve functioning. Lack of a single mineral in our food can cause mental and physical problems. We all know of the importance of calcium in our diets for building strong bones and teeth. But how many know we need manganese for the same reason?

Just as important: where are these minerals going to come from? Our soils are becoming more and more depleted of necessary minerals. Many fruits and vegetables now have fewer than 12 minerals out of the 70 plus that humans need for proper functioning - and which were present in our foods one hundred years ago. Most of us probably need some form of supplementation to supply us with all the necessary minerals for the body's optimal performance.

The truth is that some foods just aren't worth eating as food. Our physical well-being more directly depends on the minerals we take into our systems than on calories or vitamins or the precise proportions of starch, protein or carbohydrates.

You'd think, wouldn't you, that a carrot is a carrot? That one carrot is about as good as another as far as nourishment is concerned? But it isn't. One carrot may look and taste like another and yet be lacking the particular minerals our body system requires and which carrots are supposed to contain.

We know that vitamins are complex chemical substances needed for proper nutrition and that each of them is important for normal function of many special structures in the body. Out of balance conditions and disease may result from vitamin deficiencies. It's not commonly realized, however, that vitamins control the body's appropriation of minerals, and in the absence of minerals they have no function to perform. Lacking vitamins, the system can use minerals, but lacking minerals, vitamins are useless.

Metabolism, enzymes, and amino acids

In order for the body to draw valuable nutrients from the food that we eat, it is necessary for the food to be properly digested and metabolized. Digestive enzymes do the work of digestion. Unfortunately, once again, our modern life-styles are having a negative impact on important enzymes. Enzymes are extremely sensitive to heat and are destroyed by temperatures above 50 degrees Celsius (122 degrees Fahrenheit). Because we cook (and often over-cook) our foods, we need to eat more raw vegetables and fruits and supplement our intake of enzymes.

Finally, in order for the body to use the food that we eat, the body needs amino acids to make up its necessary proteins. The twenty amino acids within proteins exhibit a remarkable chemical versatility.

Of those twenty amino acids, our bodies can produce only ten. The others must be supplied in the food we eat. Failure to obtain enough of even one of the ten essential amino acids, those that we cannot make, results in degradation of the body's proteins—muscle and so forth—to obtain the one amino acid that is needed. Unlike fat and starch, the human body doesn't store excess amino acids for later use. So amino acids must be in the food every day.

Want a quick list? Amino acids we can produce are alanine, asparagine, aspartic acid, cysteine, glutamic acid, glutamine, glycine, proline, serine and tyrosine. Tyrosine is produced from phenylalanine, so if the diet is deficient in phenylalanine, tyrosine is required as well. Essential amino acids are arginine (required for the young, but not for adults), histidine, isoleucine, leucine, lysine, methionine, phenylalanine, threonine, tryptophan, and valine.

Strangely enough, the proteins the body uses aren't obtained directly from the food we eat. Dietary protein is first broken down into amino acids, which the body then uses to build the specific proteins, hormones, antibodies and neurotransmitters it needs.

The human body is a complete pharmacy. Luckily for us all, if one of the elements in that pharmacy is in short supply, a supplement can restore the balance.

The famous homeopath, Constantine Hering, made a clear distinction between the symptoms of a disease crisis and those of a healing crisis. Hering's Law of Cure: "All cure starts from the head down, from within, out, and in the reverse order that the symptoms appeared throughout the person's life."

What's the significance of knowing Hering's Law of Cure? It codifies the difference between "healing" and "disease."

CellFood® and its place in the food chain

CellFood® is a proprietary formulation containing 78 ionic/colloidal trace elements combined with 34 enzymes, 17 amino acids, and dissolved oxygen, all suspended in a solution of Deuterium Sulfate [D2S04].

The body perceives CellFood® as normal healthy body fluid, and allows the nutrients in CellFood® to pass immediately through the sensitive membranes of the mouth, throat and esophagus directly into the bloodstream. What's remarkable about CellFood® is its ability to generate new oxygen and hydrogen right within the body.

Water molecules are held together by simple attraction - one negatively-charged oxygen atom and two positively-charged hydrogen atoms. That's classic H2O. CellFood® actually weakens that attraction, leaving the molecule susceptible to breaking apart. Doing so would release two atoms of hydrogen, and one atom of oxygen - all available for use by the body. The oxygen atom now can be used for countless vital processes in the body, such as irrigating, building and strengthening cells and organs; preventing inflammation, promoting osmosis, moistening lung surfaces for gas diffusion, and regulating body temperature. Then, combined with a single carbon atom, it forms carbon dioxide (CO2), which is expelled through the respiratory system.

And when this "water splitting" takes place, the released hydrogen atoms hold an enormous amount of positively charged electromagnetic energy. This means that as the immune system is being progressively boosted, it makes the body more capable of dealing with microorganisms that could be detrimental to one's health.

CellFood® works at the physical level by providing the body with essential minerals for the constitution of the physical body. It works at the electrical and electromagnetic levels by increasing the vibrational frequencies of all the body organs, boosting the immune system, and enabling the nervous system to function more effectively. It works at the biological level by enhancing natural biological processes. It works on the chemical level by supplying amino acids to the body for building protein. It's ability to supply oxygen and nutrients to the brain supports emotional and psychological well-being.

CellFood® itself does not directly cure disease. The body has been magnificently designed to do that. CellFood® provides cells with the essential building blocks needed to achieve optimal health. Though CellFood® works on priorities at deep cellular levels, some people may not experience the results they desire. In these cases, the answer may lie in how much and how often the individual is taking CellFood®.

In case you're wondering…

A key question: Is CellFood® a medicine? **Answer:** No, CellFood® is not a medicine. It's classified as a nutritional supplement.

An equally significant question: How does CellFood® differ from other oxygen products? **Answer:** Many other oxygen products tend to flood the body with oxygen, often creating dangerous oxygen free radicals. CellFood® actually bonds with these free radicals, supplying the body with usable pure oxygen, in a time-release manner, directly to the cells.

Can you overdose on CellFood®? Answer: No. CellFood® is a nutritional supplement made from natural substances. The body only uses what it needs, and eliminates the remainder through the normal channels of elimination.

A professional athlete's question: Am I cheating if I use CellFood® during sports competitions? **Answer:** No, CellFood® is made from natural ingredients, none of which are on the "list of banned substances" issued and governed by professional and amateur athletic associations.

Last question:

What if I'm taking a prescription medicine? Answer: CellFood® can be used in conjunction with other nutritional supplements or medicines because it increases the bioavailability of these other substances, enabling the body to more effectively use them. (If you are pregnant or under medical care, consult your medical practitioner before using.)

A final thought

Technically speaking, CellFood® is not a life-changing nutrient, but essential health elements all rolled into a single life-changing nutritional supplement. The reason is plain, it's one of the hardest working products I know of that has the outstanding capacity to thoroughly oxygenate our bodies.

CellFood® is not a medicine, and no medical claims are made for the treatment, prevention, cure or mitigation of disease. So obviously there are no published "clinical tests" as is the case with medicines. With medicine, there is a cause-and-effect relationship … so Medicine A will produce Effect B, and clinical tests can prove this.

Because CellFood® is a nutritional supplement it works with the body's priorities and starts working where it is most needed. So, because everyone is unique, CellFood® is specific to each individuals health experiences. CellFood® may have an important position as an advanced development for cleansing, repairing, building, balancing and energizing the human body.

CHAPTER FIVE

Colostrum

Colostrum:
The naturally-produced vaccine against auto-immune disease & aging

Most of us were brought up to believe that by drinking lots and lots of milk, we were ensured a long, strong, and healthy life. Our forefathers may have become a bit confused … about the difference between Colostrum and a mother's milk.

Life's giant kick-starter: Colostrum -- much more than milk

Before breast milk is ever produced, our first nourishment as a newborn is a liquid-gold substance, produced by the mother during the first 72 hours of a newborn's life. This life-giving nutrient is called Colostrum.

You can think of Colostrum as a hefty health insurance policy for newborns, because it positively is, quite literally, the "vaccine" that promises the newborn the beginning of a healthy life.

Colostrum gives every newborn the giant kick-start we all need to begin life on this planet. That life-giving nutrient contains thousands of compounds that jump-start over 50 processes in the body, ranging from immunity to the regeneration and growth of each and every one of our cells.

Each drop of Colostrum is filled with the promise of life: Immunoglobulins, growth factors, antibodies, vitamins, minerals, enzymes, amino acids, and other special substances designed to "prime" the body to face a lifetime of invasion by various microorganisms and environmental toxins that otherwise could destroy us.

From puberty through the twilight years:
Can we get a booster shot, please?

Wouldn't it be wonderful if we could get a quick vaccine booster of Colostrum anytime we felt sickness coming on or life slowing down? Unfortunately, life hasn't worked that way. After the giant kick-start -- we're on our own. Or are we…?

Once we've passed puberty, our bodies quit producing adequate amounts of immune and growth factors so abundant in Colostrum. It's a gradual process most of us probably don't even register until we've hit an older age. But with the loss of these factors we eventually age and die.

We all feel the effects sooner or later. As we start aging our immune systems begin to lag, our skin sags, we get sick more often, and ultimately, gravity and immune disorders take us down for the count. Of course, we don't go down without a fight. No, we don't. Today's scientists have come up with all types of solutions to keep us fit and healthy. They research plants, minerals, and chemical compounds -- all carried out in the name of health and beauty.

Yet, there are some things these plants and minerals just can't give us – purely because they don't have them to give. Those are immune factors, five major immunoglobulins (antibodies), and growth factors (which are naturally occurring proteins capable of stimulating cellular proliferation and cellular differentiation) for our nervous system, muscles, skin and bones. No plant or mineral can give us the boost power we so desperately need to ensure we have the proper supply of immune factors.

Why are these immunoglobulins and growth factors so vital to human life?

You can only imagine what would happen to us if we weren't given this natural vaccination at birth. This natural vaccination of Colostrum and its mighty load of the five major essential immunoglobulins (antibodies) gives us:

1. IgA antibodies: These are found in the nose, breathing passages, digestive tract, ears, eyes, and vagina. IgA antibodies protect body surfaces exposed to outside foreign substances. This type of antibody is also found in saliva and tears. About 10% to 15% of the antibodies present in the body are IgA antibodies. A small number of people do not produce IgA antibodies.

2. IgG antibodies: These antibodies are present in all our body fluids. They're the smallest yet most common antibody (75% to 80%) in the entire body. IgG antibodies of great importance in fighting bacterial and viral infections. IgG antibodies are the only type of antibody that can move into the placenta of a pregnant woman to help protect the baby's fetus.

3. IgM antibodies: These are the largest of the antibodies. They're found in our blood and lymph fluid and are the first antibodies to respond to infections. They also alert the other immune system cells to destroy any foreign substances. IgM antibodies comprise 5% to 10% of all the antibodies in the body.

4. IgE antibodies: These antibodies are found in the lungs, skin, and mucous membranes. They cause the body to react against foreign substances such as pollen, fungus spores, and animal dander. They may occur in allergic reactions to milk, some medicines, and poisons. IgE antibody levels are often high in people with allergies.

5. IgD antibodies: These antibodies are found in small amounts in the tissues that line the belly or chest. How they work is not clear.

Checking the levels of each type of antibody can give your doctor a clear picture of the cause of a medical problem - but what we do about it afterwards is important.

Today, the necessity of finding a hard-working natural immune booster is more significant than in past times, if only because of the ever-increasing amounts of toxins attacking our lives and our lifestyles. The air we breathe, the food we eat, and the environment in which we live all are much more toxic to our systems than they ever were before. The vital nutrients our ancestors once easily enjoyed are lost today.

Unlike other supplements that isolate and sometimes overdose the body in unbalanced ways, Colostrum has the perfect combination of immune and growth factors and has demonstrated its ability to kill bacteria and viral invaders, to stimulate tissue repair (particularly in the bowel lining), and to stimulate the use of fats for fuel and optimal cellular reproduction (anti-aging!) over and over.

> *It's true. No other substance on earth can live up to the promise of a healthy life.*

The Colostrum Booster

Evidence is conclusive: Because of its unlimited immune factors, Colostrum truly is the promise for a healthy life. Most infectious disease-causing organisms enter our bodies through the mucous membranes of the intestinal tract, so for us to remain healthy it not only is more than critical - it's crucial – that our bodies can combat disease-causing organisms such as: bad bacteria, viruses, pollutants, contaminants and allergens at the point where they attack us.

How it works

Dr. David Tyrell of England, in the year 1980, discovered and demonstrated that the antibodies and immunoglobulins contained in Colostrum defend us in two ways:

1. A high percentage of Colostrum doesn't actually absorb into the body. Instead it remains in the intestinal tract where has its best form of attack on the disease causing organisms before they penetrate our bodies and cause us to get sick.

2. The rest of the Colostrum actually penetrates and absorbs into our systems and gets distributed throughout our internal defense processes inside the body. This active combination makes Colostrum uniquely effective as an oral supplement.

Is there a viable replacement?

Surely, we can't go about collecting a mother's production of Colostrum. But there are hundreds of published reports that exist around the world stating that these immunoglobulins and growth factors can be replenished in the human body with bovine Colostrum (from cows). What scientists have discovered is this: Immune and growth factors in bovine Colostrum are identical to those found in human Colostrum - and not just identical in structure, but many times more potent.

The amount of Colostrum a mother creates for her newborn is minute compared to the cow that can produce approximately nine gallons during the first thirty-six hours after giving birth.

Bovine Colostrum mimics the composition of our own Colostrum and contains:

- All five immunoglobulins (IgG, IgA, IgM, IgD, IgE).
- Growth factors.
- Peptides.
- Lactoferrin.
- Vitamins and minerals.

More important for us: Bovine Colostrum has a higher concentration of immune factors than human Colostrum, including as much as 40 times the IgG (the smallest but most common antibody that comprise up 75% to 80% of all the antibodies in the body) found in human Colostrum.

Even greater news: An abundance of research shows that the immune and growth factors in Colostrum are transferable between mammal species, meaning that the IgG and other antibodies in bovine Colostrum are available to humans as a viable immune booster.

Few natural supplements have the volumes of medical research that bovine Colostrum has to support its use. More than 4000 scientific papers line the medical journals with documentation of Colostrum's ability to beneficially affect a wide variety of health conditions.

Benefits include fighting off a huge menu of chronic autoimmune disorders such as:

- Sinusitis.
- Chron's disease.
- Addison's disease.
- Cystitis and yeast infections.
- Autoimmune diseases.
- Chronic fatigue syndrome.
- Fibromyalgia.
- Multiple Sclerosis.
- Lupus.
- Rheumatoid arthritis.
- Digestive disorders.
- Respiratory ailments.
- Heart disease.
- Depression.
- Resistance to colds.

If we're consistent with supplementing our bodies with Colostrum, it can continually regenerate and rebuild our entire adult bodies.

The natural vaccine against autoimmune disorders

Until recently, autoimmune diseases have been somewhat of a mystery to most health care professionals. The only recourse was to recommend treatments that simply allowed minor relief of pain and other systems. But these methods didn't counteract the bigger picture – and that is: How do you "turn-off" the immune response that caused the damage?

How do we contract autoimmune disorders?

"Leaky Gut Syndrome" seems to be the biggest culprit and one of the most common of all immune system diseases and a common denominator leading to other immune disorders.

Leaky Gut Syndrome is caused by inflammation of the gut lining brought about by antibiotics, alcohol, caffeine, contaminated foods, chemicals, and an overabundance of refined sugars.

This causes in an extreme amount of mineral loss because various carrier proteins needed to transport minerals from the intestine to the blood are damaged by inflammation. A "leaky gut" has an abnormal level of intestinal permeability, which lends itself to the propensity for proteins to be absorbed before they can be broken down. The immune system doesn't recognize these proteins and sees them just as any other invader, so it begins to make antibodies to fight the invaders.

So instead of these proteins being used to aid the body, they now present a health risk. The immune system then becomes what's called an overactive immune system. The overactive immune system is a warning sign and a precursor to contracting a number of autoimmune diseases. Colostrum can take hold of this overactive immune system and bring it down to normal levels.

Notes about Overactive Immune Systems:

In 1983, Polish researchers discovered a small protein chain called Polyprotein-rich Peptide (PRP) in Colostrum. This immune factor regulates the immune system. PRP stimulates T-cell precursors to form helper T-cells, prompting the immune system into action against pathogens. What's even more impressive is this: PRP is able to "turn off" the immune system. It does this by telling the T-cell precursors to produce T-suppressor cells. These are the cells that slow down an overactive immune response, thereby stopping the attack on the body's own tissue.

What happens when your immune system begins to turn deadly? Protein from food that was previously harmless now triggers a potentially serious allergic reaction. The results become devastating, affecting different parts of the nervous systems by destroying the membrane that covers and protects the body's nerves. The results are any number of symptoms such as memory loss, headaches, poor concentration, irritability, blurred vision, staggering gait, numbness, dizziness, slurred speech, and even paralysis.

Leaky Gut Syndrome is almost always associated with autoimmune disease. So reversing the direction of an autoimmune disease depends on healing the lining of the gastrointestinal tract. Since immune and growth factors in Colostrum don't break down during the digestive process, those factors are able to work magic inside the intestines, combating the effects of Leaky Gut

Syndrome. Colostrum growth factors are also anti-inflammatory and play a huge role in treating a leaky gut, as well as repairing damaged cells and keeping the mucous layer of the intestines sealed and impermeable to toxins.

Thus, not only can Colostrum tone down an overactive immune system, but its components can help cure an already contracted autoimmune disorder - in particular, those with inflammation of some vital organs.

Here's what clinical studies have shown

As stated earlier, the anti-inflammatory properties implicit in Colostrum have helped those who suffer from rheumatoid arthritis and Crohn's disease. It seems Colostrum has therapeutic value in treating autoimmune diseases through its immunomodulatory effects and may be able to stimulate the formation of specific suppressor cells which inhibit the development of these diseases.

Another clinical study showed that patients suffering from multiple sclerosis were given bovine Colostrum. The results: significant improvement in their condition versus those who weren't given Colostrum.

New cancer findings:

Studies showed that lactoferrin, one of the principal proteins found in Colostrum, might actually prevents colon, bladder, tongue, esophagus, and lung cancers and lung metastasis in animal models, while it's shown to shrink a variety of cancers as well. The underlying mechanisms are under study but appear to be related to lactoferrin's ability to boost immune system function. The milk fats found in Colostrum have been shown to be anticarcinogenic as well.

The solution to many of our woes... A healthy boost of Colostrum

Besides the protective benefits of Colostrum on our immune system, costly anti-aging clinics have caught on to the impressive anti-aging qualities of Colostrum. It seems that isolating and synthesizing the growth factors in Colostrum as an anti-aging supplement result in recharging us with more energy, elevated moods, smoother skin, improved eyesight, better digestion, and, yes, weight loss.

Even for the healthy individual or the athlete in training, Colostrum supplementation enhances the efficiency of amino acid and carbohydrate fuel uptake, a function within the intestines that causes more nutrients to be available for muscle cells and other vital tissue and organs. The more efficient uptake of nutrients delivers a boost in energy.

The most profound benefit, however, is the ability for Colostrum to heal Leaky Gut Syndrome, flush toxins and improve nutritional absorption. We can help out by eating a fiber/nutrient-rich diet, and giving ourselves the Colostrum booster we need to keep our immune system in tiptop shape.

CHAPTER SIX

Cordyceps

Alice's Adventures in Wonderland:
The healing properties of the caterpillar and the mushroom

You might remember Lewis Carroll's legendary story: Alice's Adventures In Wonderland. Alice's adventures opened her life to unimaginable magical places.

If you remember, along her journey Alice met the wise old smoker-caterpillar that wryly asked her: "Who are you?" Alice just wondered what the caterpillar was smoking... Maybe she should have been more inquisitive and asked right back: "Who are you?"

His answer would have amazed her: This wise old caterpillar's family tree quite possibly could've been traced to the long line of caterpillars cited since 1757 AD to carry a number of healing fungal agents on their backs, bound for the trees – those fungi readying to transform themselves into a powerful natural medicine.

Who are these caterpillars and their fungal little friends? They have been aiding people in the fight against respiratory diseases, immune dysfunctions, and a host of other properties for centuries. This is no fairy tale and no fantasy. It's real.

Unbeknown to Alice – but known to the Asians for thousands of years -- these fungal friends hitch a ride upon the caterpillar's back and together they weave that potent medicinal cure-all called Cordyceps. The beneficial end-product of the caterpillars' journey? Restoring imbalances in the body by stimulating the immune system, increasing energy and vitality, and lengthening longevity.

What are Cordyceps? They're an extremely rare medicinal mushroom-like fungus that attach themselves to the backs of the caterpillars. These fungi then take over the ride and steer their caterpillars to the trees. Instead of metamorphosing into moths, the fungi takes full rein of the caterpillar, feeding on the nutrients of the caterpillar and transforming themselves into a fruiting body of life-giving nutrients.

Discovered in the mountainous wild at elevations above 11,000 feet in isolated areas of Southwestern China, Nepal, and Tibet, Cordyceps have been used for treating circulatory, respiratory, and immune system disorders in traditional Chinese Medicine for the past 1500 years.

Cordyceps: Folklore or Fact?

Alice, of course, will go down in the annals of time as one of literature's most imaginative tales. But Cordyceps are hardly a folktale; rather, they're extraordinary jewels among supplements, for centuries considered the precious diamonds of medicinal plants used in Chinese herbal medicine. Cordyceps are major players in the role of our health; one we're most interested in knowing about because of its positive effects on our circulatory, respiratory, and immune systems as well as the liver, kidneys, and sex organs.

In the 1970's, when China opened its doors for business with the Western world, what followed was worldwide awareness of the benefits of Traditional Chinese Medicine and the demand for herbal medicines.

Some consider Cordyceps possibly the, most significant discovery for the Western World because Cordyceps specifically benefit those who suffer from:

- Emphysema
- Asthma
- Chronic bronchitis
- Cardiac arrhythmia
- Chronic heart failure
- Liver disorder
- Renal dysfunction
- Lymphoma
- Leukemia
- Impotence
- Reproductive dysfunction

The chemistry holds the key.
(We just don't know which part.)

What's truly responsible for the complex physiological actions reported? The actual active components of Cordyceps are unresolved.

Seven classes of natural chemical constituents are found in wild Cordyceps, including proteins; peptides; the entire scope of essential amino acids, polyamines, saccharides, and sugar derivatives; sterols; nucleosides (including adenine, uracil, uridine, guanosine, thymidine, and deoxyuridine); fatty acids and other organic acids; and to top off this unbelievable cocktail of beneficial ingredients, vitamins B1, B2, B12, E, and K.

Cordyceps contain twenty-eight saturated and unsaturated fatty acids. Polar compounds of wild Cordyceps extracts and manufactured Cordyceps Sinensis–4 (a strain of the wild Cordyceps) include many compounds of hydrocarbons, alcohol, and aldehydes.

In 1994, renowned UK researcher Dr. David Pegler and his colleagues proposed that Cordycepin and Cordycepic acid (d-mannitol, and 3-deoxyadenosine) were the important active ingredients. But to this day no one is sure.

In China, more than 2000 patients with various medical disorders have been involved in clinical trials using Cordyceps Sinensis-4. The chemical and pharmacological profiles are similar to natural Cordyceps and most of the research available was completed using manufactured Cordyceps Sinensis-4.

Findings: (Don't worry about tech-words. Instead, concentrate on obvious benefits.) Cordyceps show renal protective effects, hepatoprotective effects, hypoglycemic protective effects, as well as enhanced immune system activity. The substance also is used as an adjunct to cancer treatments, improving the tolerance to the adverse effects associated with radiation and chemotherapy. Anti-inflammatory properties of Cordyceps have shown to be effective as well.

Suffice it to say, though the researchers are at odds about which components of Cordyceps actually work the magic, they all agree it works.

> *Fungus Worthy: Cordyceps Sinensis is known to the Chinese as "DongChongXiaCao" and to the Japanese as "Tochukaso."*

Cordyceps pumps up your natural killer cells

A number of studies show us that Cordyceps increase the number of "Natural Killer" cells in our bodies. Natural killer cells (or NK cells) are a major component of our immune system. NK cells play a major role in the rejection of tumors and cells infected by viruses. Cordyceps not only enhance NK cell activity in healthy individuals but we've seen it in patients with leukemia and melanoma as well. According to a study published in the Chinese Journal of Integrated Traditional Western Medicine, Cordyceps enhanced the Natural Killer cell activity of leukemia patients by 400 percent. Similar improvements of Natural Killer cell activities were found in patients with melanoma cancer.

The facts: Cordyceps power the lungs

Cordyceps help those who suffer from:

- Bronchitis
- Lung cancer
- Emphysema
- Asthma

Testimonial research:

Scientific studies demonstrate how Cordyceps alleviate the symptoms of several respiratory illnesses, including chronic bronchitis, and asthma. Here's an example:

In a double-blind, placebo-controlled study with 30 elderly volunteers, it was concluded that Cordyceps improved the maximum amount of oxygen these people were able to assimilate.

For bronchitis sufferers, research claims even greater benefits: Cordyceps increased intra-tracheal secretion in rats, and loosened phlegm, which accounts for treating cough in asthmatic patients when taken with conventional therapy along with Cordyceps (incontrovertible results reported by Y.L. Qiuo and X.C. Ma, 1993). A 68-year old man suffered from bronchitis for 18 years, causing him to cough up a lot of thick phlegm, along with attacks of night sweats, panting, dizziness, heaviness in his body, and overall low energy.

After taking Cordyceps for just 5 days, his coughing and phlegm were dramatically reduced. Within two weeks the tight feeling in his chest and his panting were completely gone. He could run slowly for 200 yards. His cough had disappeared, as had dizziness and low energy. After one month of taking Cordyceps, his lung function was normal.

Case study: Emphysema. I once had a referral who suffered from an advanced case of emphysema. She was (and rightly so) mortified by the thought of suffocating to death from lack of breathing capacity. By the time I met her, her doctor had prescribed four different medications, plus weekly breathing treatments. I suggested that she also take Cordyceps in a dose of 2 grams, three times a day. She faithfully took the daily prescribed measure for 12 months, along with her medications. After the 12 months her bewildered physician took her off both the medications and the breathing treatments. As you can imagine, her doctor not only was amazed and clueless as to why her condition didn't worsen; even more profoundly, he was amazed at how her condition improved.

The facts: Cordyceps help keep your heart ticking
Cordyceps battle:
- Chronic heart failure.
- Coronary heart conditions.
- Pneumonia.
- Cholesterol.
- Angina.

Testimonial research:
During a 26-month trial test of 64 chronic heart failure patients, researchers found that by using Cordyceps (3 to 4 grams per day) in combination with standard medical therapy, the patients significantly and positively altered their overall physical, emotional, and psychological well-being, along with experiencing improvements in the shortness of breath and fatigue, compared with the control group.

Another study shows that Cordyceps lower total cholesterol by 10 percent to 21 percent and triglycerides by 9 percent to 2percent, while increasing HDL-cholesterol (the good kind) by 27 percent to 30 percent.

Case study: Coronary Heart Disease. A 70-year-old woman suffered with a coronary heart condition for 18 years. Her EKGs showed abnormalities from arrhythmia and angina. She tried many medications without results. After taking Cordyceps for one month, all clinical symptoms were gone and her EKG showed vast improvement. After completing one treatment cycle of Cordyceps, her EKG was totally normal. Her follow-up one year later showed no signs of relapse.

Case study: Asthma, edema, and heart condition. A 42-year-old woman began Cordyceps treatment for two weeks, and most of these symptoms improved. At six months all symptoms and conditions had disappeared.

The facts: Cordyceps improve the health of your liver
Cordyceps battle:
- Hepatitis B.
- General liver dysfunctions.
- Cirrhosis of the liver.

Testimonial research:

Research written up in the China Journal of Chinese Materia Medica states that in a three month open label trial Cordyceps were effective in treating chronic active hepatitis B in 33 patients and treating 8 patients with cirrhosis. The C. Sinensis-4 supplement showed 71.9 percent improvement in a "Thymol Turbidity" test of the liver and 78.6 percent in the SGPT Test of the liver.

Case study: Cirrhosis and chronic liver dysfunction

A 36-year-old man suffering from cirrhosis and liver dysfunction was experiencing severe fatigue, rib pain, abdominal bloating, low weight, poor appetite, insomnia, low grade fever, sweating and emotional problems – whew! That's enough to kill you, and certainly enough to kill him. But after taking Cordyceps for 2 months, his abdominal bloating became less severe and he was able to eat and sleep much better. After 10 months on Cordyceps all of his symptoms vanished.

The facts: Cordyceps relieve chronic kidney disease

Testimonial research

The Journal of Administration Traditional Chinese Medicine reports that patients with chronic kidney diseases showed 51 percent improved kidney function after one month of Cordyceps treatment. This study found that the supplement reduced damages to the renal tubules and protected the sodium/potassium balance on cellular membranes of the kidneys. It showed that Cordyceps decreased chronic renal insufficiencies.

In studies of rats, Cordyceps have a proven ability to inhibit the kidneys from bleeding and showing up in the urine, and to reduce the elevation of serum creatinine.

The facts: Cordyceps inhibit growth against tumor cells

Cordyceps lessen symptoms in:
- Lung cancer.
- Tumorous growths.
- Breast cancer.
- Stomach cancer.
- Leukemia.

Testimonial Research: The clinical studies in China and Japan are astounding the Western World with their impact. Example: Fifty-nine patients with terminal lung cancer given C Sinensis-4 (2 to 3 grams per day) along with chemotherapy reduced the size of the tumors in 46 percent of the patients. Not only that, but white blood cell counts could be maintained as well.

Another example: Researchers in Japan have cited that Cordyceps enhance the general reactivity of the immune system in cancer patients.

Case study: Breast cancer. A 44-year-old breast cancer patient was getting regular treatments of chemotherapy after her breast cancer surgery resulting in the depletion of white blood cells and overall immune function. After taking Cordyceps treatment for one month, all her blood chemistry came back normal and she was able to go on with treatment.

Case study: Stomach cancer. A middle-aged man facing surgery for stomach cancer was given Cordyceps for one month before the surgery. The cancer cells shrank dramatically. His stomach surgery was postponed. Just two weeks later, the cancer cells had disappeared altogether. (Re-read this paragraph. It exemplifies the power of Cordyceps.)

Cordyceps unsurpassed energy and stamina-inducing properties make the headlines

Cordyceps add vitality by:
   • Increasing the function of the heart and lungs
   • Improving sports performance
   • Building stamina

Case study: Cordyceps drive Chinese National Sports to world breaking record.

Cordyceps made huge sports headlines in 1993 at the Chinese National Games, when a group of nine women athletes went on to shatter nine world records, including shattering the 10,000-meter record by an unprecedented 42 seconds. Each team member was given a cocktail of TCM drugs and tonics including Cordyceps. That's not too shabby when you remember that the majority of athletic records are broken only by milliseconds.

At the time all those records were falling, there was talk of banning Cordyceps from sporting events as giving the user an unfair advantage. Even today, most professional athletes who use it are unwilling to admit it due to the possibility of banning the stamina-inducing mushroom. But the Canadian Olympic Committee has taken an official and logical stand and has ruled that it will be allowed in professional competition.

Since then, several reports and studies have been completed to determine the effects of Cordyceps on human performance. A study published in the Medicine & Science in Sports & Exercise Journal, 2001, concluded that Cordyceps support normal fat mobilization and beta-oxidation, preserving glycogen during prolonged exercise. It improves the flow of blood in the body by relaxing the smooth muscles of the blood vessels so it's easy for them to expand. So it's only logical to conclude that Cordyceps improve the functioning of the heart and lungs.

Not only for sufferers of disease...
We obviously can conclude that if athletes can benefit from using Cordyceps ... why shouldn't you?

Cordyceps may make a lot of medicinal claims for just one simple substance; but after long years of successful use, modern Western science has finally discovered its benefits. Due to its rarity, Cordyceps harvested in the wild are extremely expensive. Despite its cost, Chinese medicine claims that the medicinal uses of Cordyceps have made it the key ingredient for all natural remedies.

The commercialization of C. Sinensis-4 has helped make it more affordable to the general population. So at last we can all benefit from its medicinal properties.

CHAPTER SEVEN

Enzymes

Enzyme Therapy: What it means for you

Simple (maybe over simplified!) description: enzymes are catalyst-substances that cause a chemical reaction to move faster.

For example, air is a catalyst for fire. You can make the fire in a fireplace burn faster by fanning it. The parallel: Enzymes are the catalysts of biochemical reactions in living organisms. Without enzymes, these reactions would occur far too slowly for proper metabolism.

Your typical energy bar contains vitamins, minerals and sugars. Sure, energy exists in the nutrients in the bar, but those nutrients have to be unlocked before your body can utilize them. A random chemical process could take years to break down the nutrients in the bar and release the energy. A catalyst can speed this process up quite dramatically by reducing the amount of energy necessary to start releasing energy.

Enzymes 101

Enzymes are made up of amino acids. They aren't alive, nor are they living cells; so they can't die. They either become "inactive" or they become "denatured." When inactive, the enzyme is not acting on, catalyzing or digesting anything. This may be due to a lack of water, an incompatible temperature or an incompatible pH (acid/alkaline range). Enzymes are sensitive to their surroundings and when exposed to temperature or pH extremes they may become denatured. That means an enzyme loses all activity and can no longer serve as a catalyst under any condition.

Science has so far been able to identify and name over 5,000 enzymes that our bodies manufacture and utilize, but there may be far more, perhaps tens of thousands of different enzymes within the body. Why are there so many enzymes? Each enzyme has a specific job and it can do nothing other than what it is designed to do.

Digestive Enzymes

The digestive process wouldn't be possible without, catalysts with biological activity. In the digestive system this biological activity or "energy" is what enables the enzymes to break down or digest proteins, fats and carbohydrates into their simplest components (amino acids, essential fats and sugars). Enzymes also assist in the extraction of vitamins and minerals. Then the beneficial components are delivered to the trillions of cells throughout the body, while those that aren't essential or toxic are escorted out of the body.

Since digestive enzymes are responsible for this process, it is safe to say that without them, all of us would die of malnutrition. To better understand this process let's look a little deeper into digestion itself.

You've seen an apple going "bad" because it sat in the kitchen fruit bowl too long. You didn't eat it, so it ate itself. It deteriorates in front of your eyes. The enzymes within that apple have become active in a digestive manner and the result is a spoiled apple. If you want to speed that process up, simply damage the apple in any way. The soft spots on apples are damaged areas where enzymes are particularly active because they have been released from within the apple's cells … and the apple is now being digested. When we chew the apple, we are literally speeding up the reaction we have watched in our kitchen fruit bowl. If that same apple were used in an apple pie, or in a stewed apple dish, the enzymes would be denatured and of no use to us digestively. So when we eat a cooked apple, the digestive system is called on to produce the enzymes needed to digest the cooked food.

Metabolic Enzymes

Metabolic enzymes are enzymes produced within the body that aren't used for digestion. They have been called the spark of life, the energy of life, and the vitality of life because without these enzymes we would not be able to hear, feel, think, walk, talk, breathe or live.

Every organ, every tissue, and all 100 trillion cells in our body depend upon the reaction of metabolic enzymes and their energy. All living cells produce metabolic enzymes, although the pancreas, liver and gallbladder play a vital role in determining the amount of metabolic enzymes the body is capable of producing. Ah, but enzymes responsible for every function of the body cannot be produced in a lab, encapsulated, bottled, and sold to the consumer. If they could, the metabolic enzyme pills would be in every health food store and pharmacy in the world and would be responsible for curing nearly every disease.

Without enzymes, life would be impossible. Yes, a lack of enzymes is the cause of most disease, which leads to death. If you want to stay healthy, you need to support the body's mechanism for producing and conserving enzyme production. Fact: Most diseases known to man are the result of an enzyme imbalance.

Cancer cells are surrounded by a protein that protects it by disguising it from the immune system. Proper enzymes break down that protein and digest the cancer or expose the cancer to the immune system for removal. These enzymes may have a similar effect on viruses and bacteria that cause sickness since bacteria are made up of protein and viruses are protected by them.

Plant-Based Enzyme Therapy

Plant-based enzymes represent about 80% of all of the enzymes sold in health food stores. (The other 20% is made up of combination plant and animal enzyme products.)

Benefits of plant-based enzymes: The enzymes are vegetarian and vegan and can thus be consumed by everyone; they are the highest potency source, between 10 and 100 times more effective at digesting proteins, fats and carbohydrates per milligram than animal enzymes; the pH range is broad, making them active in stomach acid and throughout the rest of the body.

You can see why plant-based enzymes are usually the first choice.

Enzyme Therapy

The most obvious use of enzymes to overcome a health issue or symptom is to use them to enhance digestion. Whether a person has indigestion, heartburn, acid reflux, gas, bloating, and fatigue after eating, food cravings and the like, that person can benefit from enzymes with meals, because many of these symptoms are the result of inefficient digestion.

Any of the symptoms described is an indication that an enzyme deficiency exists. For some reason the body can't keep up with the demand placed upon it and the lack of digestive enzyme production leads to common digestive complaints. If those symptoms are left unchecked, they can lead to more serious digestive problems and a host of diseases.

Digestion and Health

By some estimates, 80 percent of the energy we use in our lifetime is used to digest the foods we eat. Yes, 80 percent. Completely digesting the average meal, from the time the food enters the body until the waste leaves, takes an average of three days. This means that every minute of every day we are digesting foods. Not a second passes that our digestive system is not working at breaking down foods, delivering nutrients and expelling waste.

What is the other 20 percent of our energy being used for? The answer is everything else. All the systems of the body including the immune, respiratory, reproductive, cardiovascular, nervous, and muscular systems share this remaining 20 percent. The digestive system consumes four times more energy per day than all other systems combined. This is why digestive symptoms are often the first clue that something is wrong with our bodies.

When we're feeling sick, although we might not have an appetite, before long we realize it already is 2:00 in the afternoon and we haven't eaten anything yet. So we eat whatever is in the refrigerator, and think we're doing the right thing.

Instead, we need to consider eating foods that require little effort from the digestive system and ones high in nutrition. Freshly juiced fruits and vegetables are a great choice during times of illness. This is precisely why fasting is so beneficial to us and promotes healing. Imagine the energy you are giving back to the body by fasting. Calorie restriction allows more metabolic energy by reducing the demand for digestive energy. Many believe this abundance of metabolic energy is the mechanism for the success of the longevity diet.

Raw food is also an option to return energy to the body. Since raw foods are full of enzymes, the enzyme content spares the pancreas from having to manufacture an excessive amount of digestive enzymes, providing more energy for other systems.

So what does this mean? If you want to stay healthy or get healthy you need to free up as much digestive energy as you can spare. This allows all the other systems of the body to have energy they need to function properly. Fasting, restricting calories, eating more raw food or taking high potency plant-based digestive enzymes at every meal can facilitate this.

Therapeutic (Systemic) Enzymes
The difference between digestive enzymes and therapeutic enzymes (or what some people call systemic enzymes) is timing.

Taken at the beginning of a meal, the enzymes assist the digestive process. Taken apart from meals on an empty stomach, they are considered to be therapeutic.

For therapeutic enzymes to have a healing effect, it is imperative that there is not a large demand for digestive energy 24 hours a day, 7 days a week. When used therapeutically on an empty stomach, the enzymes aren't digesting food; they are absorbed into the blood and can have a therapeutic effect on different systems of the body.

Why we get sick

Traveling on airplanes is a great place to get sick. We all breathe the same recycled air. If someone happens to have a cold or virus that is airborne, we are exposed to it. Though everyone on the plane is exposed, not everyone will get sick. Why would some people exposed to an airborne virus get sick and others don't? The short answer is that some people lack the metabolic enzymes needed to maintain their optimum health when they are exposed to a virus or bacteria, they get sick.

The reason so few know or write about metabolic enzymes is because the metabolic enzymes we lack cannot be placed in a pill. But even though we may not be able to replace the enzymes we are specifically deficient in with enzyme supplements, we can supply the body with what it needs to support the deficiency and thereby assist it in getting back to manufacturing the lacking enzymes.

Therapeutic Enzyme Supplements

Not many companies specialize in enzyme supplements. A few that do are Enzymedica, Theramedix, Tyler, Enzyme Research, Transformation, and Mucos Pharma. Of these companies, only a few provide supplemental enzymes exclusively. Most have an extensive line of vitamins, minerals and herbal blends combined with enzymes. One of the reasons why Enzymedica and Theramedix are among the exceptions is because the market is relatively small for such products. Since so few individuals understand the concept of enzyme therapy, only a small number of consumers will ever purchase a product made up exclusively of enzymes.

None of these companies provide metabolic enzyme products. Instead, they use plant-based, plant and animal enzymes in their formulas designed for taking apart food to be absorbed in the bloodstream.

The enzyme therapist tries to determine what category of enzymes will address the most obvious deficiency, producing the fastest results. We always start with digestion first, so the initial recommendation is to take digestive enzymes with every meal while increasing the amount of raw food consumed daily.

Suppose arthritis is present. Here we need an enzyme blend that is primarily proteolytic (one that breaks down protein) since proteases are known to reduce inflammation on many levels. Though this may sound a bit confusing, let's attempt to simplify it by outlining the most popular enzymes and their primary uses in alphabetical order.

Ready?

- **Alpha-Galactosidase** breaks down carbohydrates, especially helpful with raw vegetables and beans.
- **Amylase** (Carbohydrase) Breaks down carbohydrates, such as starch and glycogen, regulates histamine when taken on an empty stomach, reduces food cravings, and increases blood sugar.
- **Bromelain** breaks down protein and is the most beneficial as an anti-inflammatory.
- **Catalase** acts as an antioxidant by breaking down hydrogen peroxide into water and oxygen.
- **Cellulase** breaks down cellulose and chitin, a cellulose-like fiber found in the cell wall of Candida, helps free nutrients in both fruits and vegetables because of its action on the cell wall.
- **Glucoamylase** breaks down carbohydrates, specifically polysaccharides, or long chains of carbohydrates.
- **Glucoreductase** breaks down blood glucose.
- **Hemicellulase** breaks down carbohydrates.
- **Invertase** (Sucrase) breaks down carbohydrates, especially sucrose and maltose.
- **Lactase** breaks down lactose (milk sugar), used to treat lactose intolerance.
- **Lipase** breaks down lipids and improves fat utilization, helps reduce cholesterol, supports weight loss, hormone production, and gallbladder function.
- **Maltase** (Diastase, Malt Diastase) breaks down carbohydrates, malt and grain sugars, breaks down complex and simple sugars.
- **Mucolase** (non-crystalline form of seaprose) breaks down mucous, helpful for congestion and sinus infections.
- **Papain** breaks down protein, most beneficial as an anti-inflammatory.
- **Pectinase** breaks down carbohydrates, such as pectin found in many fruits and vegetables.
- **Phytase** breaks down carbohydrates, especially helpful in breaking down phytic acid found in the leaves of plants, helps with mineral absorption.
- **Protease** breaks down protein, bonds with alpha 2-macroglobulin to support immune function when taken on an empty stomach, reduces inflammation, and increases circulation.
- **Seaprose** (crystalline form of mucolase) breaks down mucous, helpful with congestion and sinus infections.
- **Serratiopeptidase** an anti-inflammatory.
- **Xylanase** breaks down soluble fiber rather than insoluble fiber.

You can readily see: The most widely researched category of enzymes are those that break down proteins, proteolytic enzymes or just proteases. When consumed with food, they assist in breaking down proteins. When consumed between meals, they are absorbed into the blood to assist with immune imbalances, heavy metal toxicity, inflammatory conditions, circulatory disorders, skin problems, constipation, water retention, inappropriate blood clots, heart disease, stroke, cancer and the like. The use of proteases for these conditions is the second most popular use of enzyme therapy, after digestive applications.

From sickness to health

The one thing that needs to be understood about illness, aside from the fact that it is the result of an enzyme deficiency, is that the cause of the illness is in some way related to protein. In order for us to stay healthy we need to be well equipped to overcome protein invaders in the body that will make us ill if left unchecked.

Here's a surprise: we are well equipped. To quote Dr. Ellen Cutler, M.D: "Our immune system is overbuilt for success." Unfortunately, we can make it under-equipped by overeating cooked and processed foods.

Help is available. We can actually supply the body with a supplement that becomes a part of the immune system.

Lipases (check out the list we just compiled) break down or disengage fat. Lipases are one of the simplest enzymes to understand and one of the easiest to recommend, as they are effective for issues related to fats. Obesity can be thought of as a deficiency in lipase. One study showed that 100% of clinically obese (over 30% their ideal body weight) individuals are lipase deficient.

Lipase is recommended therapeutically for high cholesterol, obesity, high triglycerides, heart disease, hormonal imbalances, nerve problems, fat-soluble vitamin deficiencies and skin problems such as eczema and psoriasis.

Carbohydrases are enzymes that help break down complex carbohydrates such as fruits, vegetables and legumes. Therapeutically they have been shown to regulate histamine, which is responsible for the common allergy symptoms many people experience when the pollen count in the air is high. Carbohydrases are also good at raising blood sugar. If you have sugar cravings, food cravings and low blood sugar, amylase may help tremendously. When sucrose, lactose, and maltose are not properly digested, people often exhibit symptoms that include depression, moodiness, panic attacks, manic and schizophrenic behavior, severe mood swings, abdominal cramps, and diarrhea.

If the microflora (bacteria) needed in our large intestine is out of balance, the result can contribute to many symptoms associated primarily with a condition called Candidiasis, the collection of symptoms caused by a yeast-like fungus that normally lives in healthy balance in the body.

When this balance is upset, infection results. In the mouth, it is called thrush; in the vagina, it is called vaginitis (yeast infection). Symptoms include new allergies to foods, fatigue, poor digestion, gas, heartburn, sugar cravings, irritability, frequent headaches, poor memory, dizziness, recurring depression, vaginal infections, menstrual difficulties, prostatitis, urinary tract infections, hay fever, postnasal drip, habitual coughing, sore throat, athlete's foot, skin rash, psoriasis, cold extremities, and arthritis-like symptoms.

Determining Enzyme Potency

The determining factor of an enzyme product's potency is the "effect" it has on proteins, fats and carbohydrates. In other words, the quantity of food that an enzyme can break down or digest determines its potency.

This method of measurement may differ from what most people are accustomed to. For example, when comparing two vitamin C products, the average consumer will typically compare the price and number of milligrams per tablet of one vitamin C product with another. For enzymes, it isn't as simple. Enzymes aren't measured by weight. Thus a measurement in milligrams (mg) or international units (IU) wouldn't describe the true potency of the product.

One of the key factors in determining the potency of an enzyme is the pH in which the enzyme was tested. pH is simply a measurement of acidity and alkalinity. The higher the number, the more alkaline the substance; the lower the number, the more acidic the substance. pH can range from 0 to 14 while 7 is neutral (the middle of the scale). The pH range of enzymes is an important measure of potency since it defines how long it will work in the body.

Different portions of the body function in varying pH levels. The pH of the stomach averages between 2 and 3 (very acidic), while the small intestine is alkaline at a pH of 8; the blood remains slightly alkaline at just over 7 on the pH scale. So, if an enzyme product contains a protease that has an optimal activity of 3, it will work well at digesting protein in the acid environment of the stomach, yet may not work at all in the alkaline environment of the small intestine or the blood.

Not all proteases can digest all proteins, nor can all lipases digest all fats. So the more proteases in a protease blend, the more protein it will be able to break down. Combining enzymes within categories (such as multiple proteases, lipases, amylases and cellulases) will digest or break down more protein, fat, carbohydrates and fiber, respectively. This blending also increases the range of pH the enzymes work in and illustrates how one enzyme will break less bonds and is less potent than a multiple enzyme blend.

Choosing the Right Enzyme Supplement

It's apparent that there is a lot to the science of enzyme potency. Because of this, it may be difficult for the consumer to be certain of value and efficacy when purchasing enzyme products. Few companies have the expertise needed to produce properly formulated enzyme products that truly perform as intended.

Chances are the only thing you will find of help on a supplement label is a list of the active units. Because blending the enzymes is so critical to potency, you cannot assume that the higher the active units the better the value. If you are comparing a product that costs the same price and has the same number of capsules per bottle, note whether or not one contains multiple enzymes per category.

At a health food store, you may find that enzymes are grouped together in a way that makes little sense. The bromelain and papain products are mixed in with the digestive aids and animal source enzymes (pancreatin, trypsin and chymotrypsin). You may also find detoxifying products and system cleanses on the same shelves.

Important! The key in choosing the appropriate enzyme supplement for you is to know what you are looking for. If you are looking for an enzyme formula that can help with inflammation, then you will be looking for either a bromelain, papain blend or an animal source enzyme blend. If you are trying to reduce stress digestively, you will be looking for a high potency plant-based (fungal, microbial) enzyme product.

So look for a company that specializes in enzymes. Most often you will find the best products come from companies who are not trying to be all things to everyone. Though not a lot of companies specialize in enzymes, the ones that do make very reputable and effective products.

Although potency is often difficult to assess, the best products contain high active units (not milligrams) with multiple strains in each category. Find a product with no fillers added. Many products are formulated in a way that requires fillers to be added to either fill out the capsule or help bind the tablet together.

Buy enzymes in capsules (preferably vegetarian capsules) instead of tablets. Tableting is a harsh process for enzyme products since they are more susceptible to heat and friction than ordinary vitamins. In addition, the process of tableting may also require binders or fillers.

Two companies continue to meet all of the above requirements. The first is Enzymedica, which exclusively manufactures enzyme supplements. The second company is called Theramedix and they, too meet all of the above requirements but are sold exclusively through health professionals in alternative care facilities. There are other choices that are also satisfactory as well. A few of these include: Enzymatic Therapy, Renew Life, and Garden of Life.

Conclusion

The more we come to know, the more we realize how little we know. Science has made great strides but in comparison to what we have yet to learn, we are still very ignorant as to why people get sick and what it takes to make them better. Nothing shouts that louder than science's inability to manage the common cold.

In many ways we have ignored the basics of health: diet and exercise. Modern medicine has become so involved in the science of disease and the relief of the symptoms of disease that they have turned a blind eye to the basics. In many ways biology and health have been written off as being too simplistic. Many prefer to go through life ignoring these essential elements of health and end up trying to compensate later by popping pills and taking pharmaceuticals. Don't be fooled by the beautiful simplicity of enzyme therapy: a balanced pH and the importance of good bacteria. The fact is though enzyme therapy is relatively easy to understand, there is still much we have yet to learn!

CHAPTER EIGHT

Fish Oil

Fish Oil: Arguably the most important nutritional supplement of the millennium

Grandma was right! Many baby boomers remember when their grandmothers made them take cod liver oil from a spoon to stay healthy. Today cod liver oil and other fish oils have re-emerged as one of the most important health-promoting nutritional supplements.

What's so valuable about fish oil? It's the best source of two incredibly important essential fatty acids, eicosapentaenoic acid (EPA) and docosahexaenoic acid (DHA). These are omega-3 fatty acids the human body needs to maintain health and prevent disease. But the human body does not produce enough EPA and DHA to meet its own needs. So you can see why this supplement has supreme significance.

Research and endorsements

Omega-3 fatty acids have received recognition and endorsements from the top medical organizations and policy makers in the world. Examples: American Heart Association, American Diabetes Association, World Health Organization, United Kingdom Scientific Advisory Committee on Nutrition, European Society for Cardiology, and The British Nutrition Foundation.

Scientific evidence supporting optimal intake of EPA and DHA is so prolific even the multinational food corporations are feverishly pursuing techniques to fortify food with EPA and DHA. But if your goal is to maintain health naturally, stick with Grandma's recommendations for getting enough EPA and DHA - a spoonful of fish oil.

How about taste? Fish oil has come a long way, and even Grandma would be pleased to taste it now. In three words: It tastes great. Fish oils are now available as liquids or soft gels, flavored or unflavored, and there are even chewable fish oils for kids!

From fish? Not necessarily.

The primary source of omega-6 fatty acids in the human diet is linoleic acid from the oils of seeds and grains. Sunflower, safflower, soy, and corn oil are particularly rich in linoleic acid. Evening primrose oil, borage oil, and black currant oil have a high content of the health-promoting omega-6 fatty acid.

The primary dietary source of omega-3 fatty acids is alpha-linolenic acid from seeds and seed oils derived from plants such as flax, walnuts, and canola. Lots of sources here, if properly prepared.

Metabolism of Essential Fatty Acids

The action of omega-6 is to create inflammation, while omega-3s are anti-inflammatory. The pro-inflammatory versus anti-inflammatory action of essential fatty acids is of paramount importance to human health. I'll get into that later in this chapter.

An overwhelming scientific consensus indicates that adequate intake of fish and fish oil supplements that provide preformed EPA and DHA is important for the prevention of many common chronic disease states.

A balance of Omega-6 to Omega-3 is a key to good health

We should have a typical diet that contains approximately equal amounts of omega-3 and omega-6 fatty acids. The increased availability of vegetable oils has led to a dramatic rise in the consumption of omega-6 fatty acids. Animal feeds derived from grains rich in omega-6 fats has resulted in the production of meat, fish, and eggs high in omega-6 fats and virtually void of omega-3 fats. The ratio of omega-6 to omega-3 fatty acids ranges from 15:1–30:1 (instead of the pre-industrial range of 1–2:1.)

So what? So this: A diet that provides high levels of omega-6 fats shifts the physiological state to one that promotes thrombosis, vasoconstriction, inflammation, and poor cellular health. You don't want that.

And you don't want this: Physiological changes resulting from high intake of omega-6 fats has been implicated in development of heart disease, diabetes, autoimmune and inflammatory diseases (rheumatoid arthritis, Crohn's disease, colitis, multiple sclerosis, lupus, asthma, etc.), depression, dementia, and other chronic diseases. Excess omega-6 consumption and the corresponding pro-inflammatory physiologic state is one of the most pressing public health issues of the twenty-first century.

An easy and simple change in diet

An increased intake of omega-3 fatty acids coupled with reduction in omega-6 consumption is a simple diet change could improve quality of life, reduce health care costs, and promote healthy aging.

Omega-3 modulates the "Inflammatory Response"

Inflammation isn't all bad. It's part of the body's healing process and is a normal protective mechanism. But long-term inflammation can result in chronic pain, breakdown of cartilage and muscle, increased blood clotting, increased development of atherosclerotic plaques, and genetic changes, plus chronic diseases ranging from arthritis, heart disease, ADHD, asthma, eczema, depression, to cancer.

The inflammatory response is activated when the body is exposed to trauma, allergens, toxic chemicals, or disease. And the inflammatory response causes omega-3 and omega-6 fatty acids to be released from cell membranes and quickly converted into "eicosanoids" (don't worry about that tough word) that signal the surrounding tissue to respond.

So what happens? Omega-6 fatty acids are converted into pro-inflammatory eicosanoids that promote vasoconstriction and increase blood clotting, pain, and inflammation. Omega-3 fatty acids and GLA are converted into eicosanoids that support an anti-inflammatory immune response and help the body quickly return to its proper balance.

Inflammation has been a bonanza for pharmaceutical companies. One of the most profitable drug categories throughout history, the non-steroidal anti-inflammatory drugs (NSAIDs), which includes ibuprofen, aspirin, Aleve, Bextra, the ill-fated Vioxx, and Celebrex have been designed to prevent the formation of pro-inflammatory omega-6-derived eicosanoids.

Unfortunately, long-term use studies show that many of these drugs can greatly increase the risk of stomach irritation, ulcers, heart attack, stroke, and potentially lethal stomach bleeding. A happy difference: Fish oil has been proved to be an extremely safe and effective way to lower inflammation … and thereby to prevent the diseases and ailments associated with it.

EPA, DHA, hope for Alzheimer's, and metabolizing fats

Over the past 30 years of fish oil research, the anti-inflammatory activity of fish oil has been attributed mainly to EPA. All right, then, what about DHA? From a biochemists perspective EPA and DHA are structurally similar. Both reside in the cell membrane, and both are released from the cell membrane when the immune system is triggered. Recently it has been discovered that both EPA and DHA function as a team to mitigate excess inflammation and promote health and longevity. And the team also has been shown to exhibit protective effects in animal models of stroke and of Alzheimer's disease.

More: The team seems to improve insulin function, helps metabolize dietary fats, and reduces the formation of new fatty tissue. Beyond that, EPA and DHA are particularly important for the proper development of the brain, eyes, and nerve tissue.

Want to live well beyond age 100? When it comes to living a long and prosperous life omega-3 fats again show promise. When cell membranes of centenarians (those who lived past 100) were compared to other groups, one of the main differences was higher levels of the omega-3 fatty acids, EPA and DHA, and reduced content of the pro-inflammatory omega-6 fatty acids, linoleic and arachidonic acid. So higher levels of EPA and DHA in the cell membrane shows a relationship with living longer!

Your heart and omega-3

Cardiovascular diseases, including stroke, are the number one killer in the U.S.

Clinical trials demonstrate how omega-3 fatty acids improve heart health by reducing triglyceride levels, decreasing atherosclerosis, improving arterial function, lowering blood pressure, and reducing the risk of thrombosis.

Evidence from studies tells us that taking from 500 mg to about 1,500 mg of combined EPA and DHA each day significantly reduces deaths from heart disease. The American Heart Association (AHA) recommends that Americans with existing risk factors for cardiovascular disease should consume a minimum of one gram of combined EPA and DHA per day. Individuals with elevated triglycerides need two to four grams of combined EPA and DHA daily. Because these recommendations are more than can readily be achieved through diet alone, the AHA recommends a high quality fish oil supplement.

A sound start: Make sure you get at least one gram of combined EPA and DHA per day. This is easily achieved by taking two concentrated fish oil soft gels (each soft gel should provide approximately 550 mg of combined EPA and DHA). (If soft gels are hard to swallow, try a high quality fish oil liquid.)

Find a fish oil product fresh and free from rancidity. That just means a fish oil product that tastes great.

Fish oil and the brain

DHA is important for development of the brain and nervous system in infants. As mentioned, DHA also protects and repairs the brain and nervous tissue from age-associated damage, which improves mental function and prevents dementia and Alzheimer's in the aging population. Omega-3 supplementation can improve cognitive function in infants and toddlers, as well as improve cognitive performance in individuals over 70 years of age.

And get this: EPA helps conditions associated with altered mood and behavior including depression, bipolar disorder, schizophrenia, and ADHD. Lower levels of omega-3 fats are found in individuals who suffer from depression and bipolar disorder.

Lower levels of omega-3 fats are seen in children with ADHD and children who have difficulties with learning, behavior, reading, spelling and language. Omega-3 as significantly increased language and learning skills in children diagnosed with autism and Asperger's.

So here's the scientific consensus: All adults should eat fish at least, or more than, two times per week; patients with mood, impulse control, or psychotic disorders should consume one gram of combined EPA and DHA per day; higher levels of omega-3 supplementation may be useful in patients with mood disorders; and the use of more than three grams per day should be monitored by a physician.

Fish oil's benefits during pregnancy, infancy, and breast-feeding

The fetus is dependent on its mother for DHA intake that has to be sufficient to maintain her own healthy levels and meet fetal demands, especially during the last trimester. Fish oil supplementation improves DHA status of mothers, their breast milk, and infants. Higher DHA status has been correlated with helping women get pregnant, lowering the risk of premature births, and reducing the risk of post-partum depression.

Beyond that, getting enough DHA during pregnancy may improve behavior, attention, focus, and learning in children, reduce the risk of allergies, positively influence immune development, and increase intelligence in babies and children. A Scandinavian study found that children born to mothers who had taken cod liver oil (two tsp/day) during pregnancy and lactation had higher IQs than those born to mothers who had taken the corn oil placebo. On the other end, lower brain DHA levels are associated with cognitive deficits and increased anxiety, aggression, and depression in children.

How about your eyes?

Omega-3 fatty acids from fish oil help maintain healthy structure and function of your eyes by supporting the body's natural anti-inflammatory response, enhancing tear production, and protecting eyes from oxidation- damage.

A study of more than 32,000 women showed that women who consumed more omega-3 fats experienced a significant reduction in the occurrence of Dry Eye Syndrome. Higher intake of omega-3 fats is also associated with decreased likelihood of having age-related macular degeneration and cataract.

Down to business: How much fish oil should you take?

Let's agree in front that diet should be your first source of omega-3 fatty acids. To meet the minimum recommended amount of EPA and DHA, consume a minimum of two servings of cold-water fatty fish such as salmon, sardines, herring, anchovies, or mackerel per week. That's equivalent to approximately 200 to 500 mg of combined EPA and DHA per day.

But quality fatty fish isn't a regular part of most people's diet. And a lot of the fish consumed by Americans are low in omega-3 fats. Example: farm-raised fish, fed omega-6-rich grain. So for individuals not getting enough dietary EPA and DHA it is an absolute necessity to take a fish oil supplement daily.

To achieve the documented health benefits of fish oil many experts recommend at least 200–500 mg of combined EPA and DHA daily. Professionals across several medical disciplines agree that a daily dose of one gram of combined EPA and DHA per day is required to maintain health and support the cardiovascular system, eyes, and nervous system.

That recommendation is reflected in both the American Heart Association and The American Psychiatric Association recommendations. Certainly, the millions of Americans on anti-depressants, anti-anxiety and other mood stabilizing drugs, plus those on blood pressure medications, lipid-lowering agents, and other heart medications, all should all be taking one gram of combined EPA and DHA daily.

That may not be enough. To support an anti-inflammatory response, a minimum of three grams of EPA+DHA is in order.

And not to worry. The US Food and Drug Administration (FDA) classified omega-3 fatty acids from fish oil as "generally recognized as safe." In fact, The FDA has ruled that up to 3 grams of combined EPA and DHA is safe to be included in the food supply of Americans without fear of any negative reactions. And there are no known significant drug interactions with omega-3 fatty acids. (Obviously, as is true of all nutritional supplements, tell your doctor what you are taking.) A caution: Don't combine fish oil with blood thinning medication or before surgery without a doctor's supervision.

What to look for when buying Fish Oil

Fish oil supplements vary in potency and/or ratio of EPA and DHA. There are two main types of non-concentrated fish oils. The first is typically derived from the body of smaller fish such as sardines and anchovies, and contains approximately 18% EPA and 12% DHA. The other non-concentrated fish oil is cod liver oil, from the livers of Cod, and contains approximately 14% DHA and 9% EPA. Cod liver oil also contains naturally occurring fat-soluble vitamins A and D, and those can fluctuate in concentration with the season.

Be sure your fish oil supplement is fresh. Fish oil that has been subject to oxidation may do more harm to the body than good. So if you may be taking a "commodity grade fish oil" from a discount grocery store, do a taste test. First, chew a gel such as Nordic Naturals ProOmega soft gel, and take note of the pleasant lemon flavor. Second, chew a commodity grade soft gel. Your senses can detect higher quality, fresh oil and distinguished it from the potentially rancid commodity brand. Commodity grade fish oil will typically carry the characteristic rank taste and smell of a bad fish oil product.

Don't underestimate the value of an old fashion taste and smell test. If fish oil smells or tastes rank, throw that bottle out.

It makes sense. If you ordered sushi and it smelled bad, would you eat it? Rotten fish is no different than rotten fish oil. A bad smelling and tasting fish oil is nature's way of telling us not to ingest it.

Conclusion

With all the benefits fish oil offers, this is one supplement that not only should be on your shelf; it should be in your body, every day.

This is especially true since clinical result after clinical result verifies: Only good can come from one of nature's most valuable … and most available … natural health-aids.

CHAPTER NINE

GH3

GH3 – The guarantee for prolonged youth and longevity

Being asked if he was tired after a performance, the ninety-three-year-old cellist, Pablo Casals, said, "Why should I be? I'm the same man I was fifty years ago." The New York Times, January 3, 1971.

Can we make the same claim as the famous cellist Pablo Casals? We can all agree on one thing: growing old is inevitable and often frightening. We fight it though, oh yes we fight hard. Every day we look into the mirror, and one day our vanity kicks in when we begin noticing the ever-increasing wrinkles, sagging skin, and the decline of our "oomph" and passion as life begins to tip the scales in the wrong direction.

Aside from the outward appearance of aging, the most frightening nightmare for us all, is becoming a physical derelict in our latter years, leading a life without dignity, or becoming a burden to those around us and an embarrassment to ourselves.

So, what do we do? We start grasping at straws, and most of us are willing to try just about anything and a lot of us lose our hard earned cash to false promises.

The intensity and speed of our aging process depends largely on three groups of factors:

1. Hereditary factors, contained in our chromosomes.
2. External factors, such as diet, smoking, exercise, and stress.
3. Harmful free radicals (natural waste products produced by the body, causing cell damage.)

"Time is the killer of organic substance and it puts its definite imprint on the human organism." Dr. Ana Aslan

Is it really possible to reverse the signs of aging?

The now world-renowned Dr. Ana Aslan, was the scientific director of the National Institute of Geriatrics in Bucharest, Romania and pioneer of the miracle anti-aging formula of GH3 said yes! It is possible to reverse the signs of aging.

Aslan defined growing old as a progressive decline in the function of our cells, tissue, and organs and hence a progressive decline in the function of our immune and defense systems and regenerative capacity.

In 1949 Dr. Ana Aslan discovered the substance called Procaine (an anesthetic used mainly in dentistry), which she later called GH3 after adding additional buffers to the composition. Note: She has never claimed priority over procaine, but instead has given credit to those who first investigated procaine and its effects on the human body. Her claim, which we must repeat, is that she was the first to discover the anti-aging abilities of procaine; and she proved them time and again throughout the world.

What she discovered was that this buffered formula of procaine (GH3), contained highly effective anti-inflammatory properties, stimulated the blood supply, and slowed down the human aging process.

According to Dr. Aslan, GH3 works on our bodies at the cellular level. Our bodies are made up of different types of cells (skin, muscle, brain, nerve, bone). As long as more cells are formed than are dying, we continue to grow, this process continues into the early ages of our 20's. By the time we reach our 30's we lose more cells than we form.

Once this cellular exchange becomes unbalanced, the functions of our bodies and brains start to deteriorate. This is the pivotal time when GH3 can truly make its mark. Its ability to feed, rejuvenate and replenish our cells helps combat the ravages of life. The majority of us treated with GH3 look and feel much younger than those who don't use GH3.

By the mid-1960s she had given tens of thousands shots and pills of GH3 and is quoted as saying: "We can increase our longevity, and actually reverse the physical signs of aging as well. GH3 promises to help you look and feel younger. The richer the nutrients in our food, along with GH3, the more we see the remarkable results."

The discovery
Along with many scientists, Prof. Aslan studied many aspects of the effects of GH3, after which she put together her own therapy protocols, later known as the "original ASLAN Therapies." Professor Aslan was rewarded many international scientific honors. She was head of the UNO and WHO health-commissions and spoke about her work in lectures around the world. Many universities turned to procaine research and mostly confirmed the results of Professor Aslan's lifelong work.

"Old age is full of suffering and pain and I regard this as a parasite of life which develops slowly. I declared war on aging. As a gerontologist and a geriatrician you have to explain to healthy and sick people, what it means to grow old, and what they have to do in order to improve the quality of their life. My treatment is a solution and Gerovital-H3 is not only a treatment, it is a philosophy and a hope". - Dr. Ana Aslan

How does it work?

GH3 is a formulation of procaine hydrochloride buffered and stabilized with potassium metabisulfite and benzoic acid.

Aslan found that these buffers changed the nature of the procaine from its primary use. Unbuffered procaine is too unstable to last long enough to have the effect that GH3 does.

Procaine hydrochloride is metabolized in the body, producing PABA (para-aminobenzoic acid) and DEAE (diethyl amino ethanol), which are vitamin precursors in forming folic acid, choline and acetylcholine, vitamin K and vitamin B12.

According to Dr. Aslan, GH3 in tablet form works better in the intestines to synthesize vitamin precursors partly as a result of the breakdown of GH3 into PABA and DEAE.

GH3: the "pro-vitamin"

GH3 is a compound that leads directly to the formation of vitamins in our bodies. Because of this, domestic GH3 tablets are protected for sale by the Dietary Suplements Act of 1994. As GH3 breaks down, it releases its two constituents PABA and DEAE. They, too, have an important role before they are metabolized. PABA stimulates the "good" intestinal flora to produce such needed vitamins as folic acid and vitamins K and B1. DEAE participates in the making of choline and acetylcholine, vital factors in the body (liver and spleen), brain and nerve synapses.

GH3 produces PABA and DEAE in the body, and combines them with a weak, covalent bond, allowing them to enter the cells more efficiently once produced. For this reason, taking DMAE and PABA separately or its by product DMAE doesn't produce the same results, because they don't enter the cells in their individual form.

Procaine is more than the sum of its components: neither PABA nor DEAE, used alone, possess the same attributes as procaine. By the same complex process, GH3 is far superior to ordinary procaine in its anti-aging, and anti-depressive effects.

"To grow old in a beautiful and dignified way is at the same time a science and an art." - Dr. Ana Aslan

GH3 Benefits at a glance:

- Prevents or reverses cardiovascular disease
- Prevents arthritis
- Reverses or slows the symptoms of Parkinson's disease
- Alleviates depression – GH3 acts as an antidepressant by modifying the monoamine level in the brain
- Revives energy
- Improves memory, concentration and attention
- Improves sexual function
- Lessens graying hair and baldness
- Restores youthful vigor, and improves skin, wrinkles, nails, by combating the adverse signs of cutaneous skin aging, by maintaining or enhancing the thickness of the skin, particularly the thickness of the epidermis
- Balances the endocrine system
- Reduces cortisol levels
- Increases resistance to infections
- Improves visual, audio and olfactory acuity
- Alleviates chronic diseases, chronic rheumatism, atherosclerosis, bronchial asthma psoriasis, vitiligo, and varicose ulcers
- Retards the aging rhythm and prevents chronic diseases
- And acts as a powerful antioxidant.

Skeptical? I was too. But today GH3 is a steady, and essential part of my daily diet.

The effects of GH3 on depression

Dr. Vladimir G. Jancar, a research psychiatrist was one of the first in this country to test GH3 tablets and its effects on depression. He tried GH3 on seven of volunteer patients. Dr. Jancar is quoted as saying, "I am surprised by the efficacy of the GH3 tablets. With the patients treated, GH3 proved equal, if not superior to other anti-depressant drugs."

Dr. Jancar findings:

"One of my patients was moderately depressed and arthritic, with a blood sedimentation rate of 38 (very high). She responded well to the medication, lost her depression, and after the fourth week her arthritic pain swelling of the joints disappeared. Upon completion of the course of treatment, laboratory tests showed her sedimentation rate had dropped to 8. Her maintenance level was four tablets a day for six weeks, with a two-week interruption. She also showed no side effects, such as blurred vision and constipation. On the contrary, her physiological functioning improved. In order to follow the FDA protocol, she took three tablets a day for the first two weeks, four tablets a day the second two weeks, and six tablets a day the last two weeks. The six tablets proved too much and caused palpitation, which disappeared when the medication was reduced."

GH3 the all-purpose age rejuvenator

GH3 is beneficial in treating cardiovascular diseases, arthritis, Parkinson's disease, depression, loss of energy, memory problems, sexual dysfunction, wrinkled skin, graying hair and baldness. This supplement is widely promoted as an all-purpose rejuvenation treatment that can restore youthful vigor in the elderly.

GH3 the stress-buster and endocrine balancer

Over a lifetime cortisol damages the brain, muscle, bone, skin and the immune system. The hippocampus is key regulatory center of the brain which may gradually lose 20% of its cells due to its unique sensitivity to cortisol damage. The hippocampus, a mid brain structure strategically seated above the hypothalamus/pituitary gland and below the cerebral cortex, plays a crucial role in cognition, attention, memory, emotional stability and sensory integration. It also plays a major role in regulating the hypothalamic – pituitary axis, which in turn regulates the entire endocrine system of our bodies.

GH3 reduces high cortisol levels. Cortisol is the hormone responsible for stress and one of the few hormones that increase with age.

High-cortisol levels are shown to be a leading cause of age acceleration. The reason: Cortisol "attacks" the hypothalamus, (the area of the brain that "controls" the endocrine system). Ironically, high levels of cortisol can turn on the brain causing the greatest damage to the hypothalamus, which controls the adrenal glands that produce cortisol!

What a catch-22. This vicious cycle leads to an impaired endocrine system and supports a big role in The Neuro-endocrine Theory of Aging.

The Neuro-endocrine Theory of Aging as described by Dr. Ward Dean:

"The central thesis of the Neuro-endocrine Theory is that the aging process is caused by an age-related loss of central (hypothalamic) and peripheral receptor sensitivity to inhibition by hormones and other signaling substances. This loss of hypothalamic sensitivity results in a progressive shifting of homeostasis (the body's regulatory system for maintaining internal balance) and altered levels of hormones, neurotransmitters, and cell signalers. These metabolic shifts are believed to cause aging and the diseases of aging." ~ Ward Dean M.D.

GH3 and Alzheimer's disease

The hippocampus is found to be ravaged in Alzheimer's dementia and is damaged to a lesser extent in "normal" aging. Surprisingly, it has been discovered that as the hippocampus is more and more damaged through a lifetime of stress-induced cortisol secretion, the hippocampus loses its ability to regulate cortisol secretion. GH3 is shown to safely and effectively protect the structure, function, health, and stability of the hippocampus, and at the core of promoting a healthy and vibrant middle and old age.

You'll hear the claims of opposition

Some scientists have claimed that the stabilizers in GH3 were irrelevant and unnecessary. Going on that assumption, they performed various small scale, short-term experiments using procaine alone, without the stabilizers, and found it failed to confirm Aslan's GH3 rejuvenation effects. This followed another claim that the thousands of patient years of clinical experience and multi-faceted success using GH3 to be fraud, delusion, and quackery.

Let's make a note: this is a standard method used by the medical establishment to "refute" claims they consider to be heresy.

Dr. Aslan was noted as stating: "With the passing of time I learned that the opposition made me more and more ambitious. I knew that I was right and I had to prove it. Life would be too dull without controversy, and in my case, unfortunately, the controversies overstepped the bounds of academic dispute. All this doesn't matter now, I forgave them many years ago."

When can you expect to feel the effects of GH3?

What I can say to you is this: Good things come to those who wait. As true in most cases, those of us who expect results and expect them right now, may need to find the "fine art of patience." However, most people feel the mildly euphoric effects of GH3 within 1-3 days of first taking it. For the total actions of GH3 to fully take effect, I recommend taking it for 3-6 months. It can be continued with periodic short breaks indefinitely, or repeated as a cycle once or twice a year.

I'll now repeat the same quote I made at the beginning of this chapter:

Being asked if he was tired after a performance, the ninety-three-year-old cellist, Pablo Casals, said, "Why should I be? I'm the same man I was fifty years ago." The New York Times, January 3, 1971.

Now, you too, can make the same claim as Pablo Casals.
A note of thanks to Dr. Ana Aslan who knew what she was talking about.

> "Disease can be prevented, treated, or if it becomes chronic it can be alleviated. Disease can also often hide aging and for this reason we should pay attention to the timing." GH3 – time in a bottle.

CHAPTER TEN

Hyaluronic Acid

Reclaim your youth
Your Body's Internal Bath: Hyaluronic Acid

Would you be skeptical if someone said you could restore your youthful appearance - not just superficially - but from the inside out?

The answer has to be yes. We all are skeptics to some degree. Skepticism is good … it makes us probe deeper, to get the facts. I'll tell you a secret: your body holds the ingredients to let your unique beauty keep shining outward to the world.

Anti-aging fact: Our ever-present internal "bath" keeps us vibrant.

Yes, we've all heard it before: "When you're feeling sick, you're often told to drink plenty of fluids to keep your body hydrated." But what we don't realize is how our bodies are wired to keep us cleansed from the inside out. And sometimes our bodies need help from us. Now, I'm not talking about drinking eight 8 oz. glasses of water every day (although that's extremely important as well).

Think about this: One of the biggest culprits of our aging bodies is moisture loss. We can see how fast the steady decline of our essential body fluids affects us as we start to experience sagging skin, creaking bones, stiffening joints, rigidity, dwindling height, sunken eyes, shrinking brain, and raspy voice – every one of these is due to lack of the lubricating moisture essential to keep us vibrant.

Those symptomatic signs of aging can be washed away, simply by keeping our bodies replenished with our own internal moisturizing mechanism. And that mechanism is called Hyaluronic Acid, a fluid-like gel that bathes our cells.

Hyaluronic Acid or HA is found in a subset of the polysaccharides called the glycossaminoglycans or (GAGs). Now, please don't say, "So what." You don't have to know the techno/scientific terminology to agree on the importance of this readily available supplement. Keep reading, because I'm about to explain its significance.

Anti-aging fact: Hyaluronic Acid keeps our cells cleansed.

Keeping our cells cleansed sounds important - but why? Let's take a look: Every nutrient our bodies produce has a specific role to play. When one breaks down, there's usually a backup system. But as we age this backup system can alter, creating huge havoc on all our internal systems.

Meet the GAGs family: Glycossaminolgycans are long unbranched polysaccharides (large, macro-molecules) containing what's called a repeating disaccharide unit. These units are used for storing sugars, like starch and glycogen, playing a role in the structural supports for our cells and connective tissues.

GAGs are found mostly on the surface of our cells, or extra cellular matrix (ECM). Their negatively charged molecules have a glue-like quality in its solution. Because of the high gluey properties of GAGs, they have low compressibility, which makes these molecules ideal for a lubricating fluid in our joints. At the same time their rigidity gives structural integrity to our cells and provides open passageways between cells.

HA is unique from all the other GAGs because it doesn't attach to proteins. It's individually synthesized without a protein core and instead gets spun out by enzymes at the cell surface and goes directly into the extra cellular space, skipping the protein-binding process. HA polymers are giants (molecular weights of 100,000 - 10,000,000), which make it capable of displacing vast amounts of water. This action makes HA polymers excellent lubricators and shock absorbers.

More good news: Since HA skips protein attachment as a proteoglycan; it doesn't run the risk of faulty work if the proteins in our bodies become altered. As we discussed previously in our discussion of Carnosine: When we age our proteins are at risk of becoming altered by Advanced Glycation End Products (an apt acronym – AGES), cross-linking with glucose, all of which make proteins destructive once we stop producing large amounts of Carnosine (refer to page 31-40).

Our extra cellular matrix ECM essentially keeps our skin, bones, cartilage, tendons, and ligaments supported because of the Hyaluronic Acid it contains. This matrix is made up not only of HA, but fibrous elements called, elastin, proteins, proteoglycans, and collagen, that give our cells structure. About 3000 milligrams of HA is produced daily in the human body by specialized cells called fibroblasts (the most common cells found in connective tissue).

> *Fact: Hyaluronic Acid is fast becoming the exceptional nutrient as a biomaterial bridge in tissue engineering research.*

Anti-aging fact:
Hyaluronic Acid's crucial role in keeping our bodies young

Imagine this: If it weren't for Hyaluronic Acid our bodies would be shapeless without this invaluable fluid-like glue HA bathes us in. Here's why: HA can be found in every tissue of our bodies.

The main function of HA is replenishing and moisturizing these collagen and elastin fibers with nutritious water-based fluid. This fluid keeps the collagen and elastin fibers from overstretching (sagging) and drying out. And this fluid wouldn't even exist if the HA molecule wasn't capable of miraculously binding up to 1000 times its weight in water. That's why scientists liken HA to cement, or to the mortar needed to lay bricks.

When we're young, our skin has high levels of HA. Unfortunately levels of HA deplete as we age. An example: Think about a baby's skin – it's smooth, pliable and wrinkle-free. Compare this to an elderly person, where the skin is thinner, more wrinkled – all due to lower levels of HA as we age.

Ensuring healthy youthful skin and joints can only come from the inside out. By replacing the Hyaluronic Acid that begins depleting as we age, we can actually help reverse the signs of aging and keep our bodies running like the well-oiled machine it was made to be.

The benefits of Hyaluronic Acid:

- Lubricates your bones and joints.
- Helps keep your skin youthful and wrinkle-free.
- Retains essential fluids in your eyes.
- Maintains and supports healthy skin, scalp, lips, and gum structure.
- Nourishes your tendons and ligaments by increasing body hydration and removing waste.
- Builds strong cartilage from heart valves to the cartilage surrounding the joints.
- Keeps your blood vessels strong and flexible.

In essence, Hyaluronic Acid replenishes the internal moisture we need so desperately to keep our bodies fluid, flexible, and youthful.

Anti-aging fact:
Hyaluronic Acid - the moisture that binds our youth

Let's face it: If you've reached the age of 40, you're probably experiencing the beginning of at least one of these symptoms of aging: joint pain, wrinkles, sagging skin, and slow healing. If you're not over 40, pay close attention because we all wind up there.

Most scientists will tell us the biggest common denominator of aging is the degeneration of our connective tissue that supports the cells (which in turn accounts for lost production in HA as well). Connective tissue is found everywhere in your body. It binds the bones, muscles and skin. But it does much more than just connect muscle to bone and bone to bone. The connective tissue has three basic structural elements:

1. Ground substance (Hyaluronic Acid)
2. The stretchy fibers: (collagen and elastin).
3. Plus, a cell type.

Connective tissue is actually made up of the first element – the ground substance Hyaluronic Acid. Here's how it works on connective tissue: HA separates and cushions the cells of the connective tissue, giving them the ability to bear weight, take tension, and bounce back from abuses of the body. That is exactly how HA keeps us from falling apart at the seams: Its gel-like fluid binds the connective tissue to bones, muscles and our skin.
The benefits of supplementing your body's own production of HA to

rejuvenate the skin and protect the joints are well demonstrated. But don't forget its great potential as an anti-aging agent and as a compound that can help maintain proper immune system function.

An astounding example is Yuzurihara, Japan: The "village of long life"

Yuzurihara, Japan is vastly well known to researchers as the "village of long life." You'll find people living to advanced ages (10 times as many people live past the age of 85 as is true of the United States) without signs of wrinkles or typical age-related diseases. The researchers found that some adults (even life-long smokers!), including those who had worked outdoors, exposed to the sun day-in and day-out for most of their lives, had virtually no wrinkles -- and Yuzurihara never has had a recorded case of skin cancer.

The town's people age healthier, enjoy greater joint mobility, superb vision, and unusually smooth and well-toned skin. Health authorities attribute their youthful features to their unique diet.

Unique? You can share this diet. The secret: Hyaluronic Acid. HA is constantly replenished from foods found in the local Yuzurihara diet of sticky vegetables.

Anti-aging Fact: Hyaluronic Acid replenishes and firms your skin

Fifty percent of our entire storage of Hyaluronic Acid is found inside our skin. Its sole function: to retain structure and moisture to the inner layers of the epidermis as well as the epidermal top layers, working its magic by zeroing in at the cellular level.

HA regulates the life cycle of our skin cells.

Not only does HA penetrate deep into the dermis and hypodermis layers of our skin but it works its way up the to the outer epidermis layer of our skin, transporting nourishing molecules and eliminating pollutants and metabolic waste products for our upper cells to thrive. You can see how it plays a vital role in regulating the life cycle of our skin cells.

It's also the key ingredient that supports, forms, nourishes and hydrates collagen fibers. When collagen fibers become altered, our skin tone and elasticity dries up and becomes brittle, much like a rubber band drying out and breaking, leaving us with – yes – wrinkled sagging skin. When Hyaluronic

Acid stops producing in our tissues the weakened HA begins to trickle like a leaky faucet rather than lathering our skin with its internal lubricating fluid. From then on, the skin gets thinner, dried, tough, saggy, and wrinkled. It's easy to envision the difference: If the collagen fibers were constantly bathed in water the chances of these fibers drying out and breaking is nil. HA is the "watering system" that keeps the collagen moist and elastic.

You may have heard from your pharmacy or even experienced: The ability of Hyaluronic Acid to retain water and moisture makes it a popular ingredient in high-end cosmetic moisturizers as well. Taken internally by injections, it helps to increase skin moisture, smoothness, and firmness at and around the injection site.

> *Skin-worthy note: HA protects the skin from those nasty and ravaging free radical groups. When our skin is exposed to UVB and UV rays, it gets sunburned and the cells in our skin stop producing as much HA, while increasing the rate of collagen degeneration. HA supplements to the rescue, by scavenging free radicals.*

Anti-aging fact:
Hyaluronic Acid fends off the crippling effects of aging joints

The most common age-related crippler for people today is debilitating joint pain and muscle pain. To prove it, thousands of prescriptions are written every day, just to relieve stiffness and pain due to the deterioration of our joints and bones.

HA is a major component of cartilage.
The most familiar variety of cartilage found in our bodies is hyaline cartilage, formed throughout our skeletal system. Hyaline cartilage covers the long bones where bending occurs and provides a cushioning effect for our bones. It's also known as "gristle cartilage" because it resists wear and tear.

Our joints are surrounded by synovial fluid. This precious fluid forms capsules around the ends of two articulating bones. It secretes a liquid, a thick fluid, and it works as a shock absorber for the joints and to carry nutrients to the cartilage. Because cartilage doesn't have blood flow it relies on Hyaluronic Acid to do the job.

Thousands of people who otherwise might have to endure knee replacements are walking, running, and playing tennis because their alert physicians have given their knees injections – of Hyaluronic Acid.

Take a look:
- HA is one of the best lubricants and shock absorbers found in nature.
- HA stimulates the growth of cartilage in our joints.
- HA suppresses PGE2 (a hormone like chemical responsible for producing inflammation) production to stop pain and inflammation of joints, by hydrating and lubricating the synovial cell membrane.
- HA provides antioxidant support to prevent and reduce inflammation.
- HA is a powerhouse in fighting against connective tissue disorders, such as osteoarthritis, rheumatoid arthritis, and fibromyalgia.

Bone-worthy: People with signs of premature aging and connective tissue disorders might be able to trace their symptoms to nutritional deficiencies, often the very nutritional factors that influence the production of Hyaluronic Acid. It's been documented that people with connective tissue disorders have low amounts of Hyaluronic Acid in their bodies.

Yes, infinite amounts of prescription medicines are making millions of dollars for the pharmaceutical companies, touting relief of joint pain (many of these prescription formulae associated with long term side-effects). However, there are plenty of natural remedies that are just as effective, if not more – and with no side effects. Applications of HA, like NLHA (an oral preparation of Hyaluronic Acid), are a strategic move toward natural therapies becoming more mainstream.

The main benefit of supplementing our own bodies with Hyaluronic Acid has been well researched. Scientists have discovered that Hyaluronic Acid taken orally is an essential to maintain the skin, joints, and eyes.

Anti-aging fact: Hyaluronic Acid keeps your eyes focused

HA along with water (about 99% of the total volume of vitreous is water) forms the bulk of the vitreous humor, the stable gel in the eyeball that fills the space between the lens and the retina. Since HA was discovered in the vitreous, it has been used as a lubricant in eye surgery.

HA is often used as a lubricant for the corneal epithelium, helping in the growth and migration of cells across the cornea, making it one of the effective healing agents for any eye wounds and tissue regeneration in the eye.

As previously discussed in this chapter, thin fibrils give structure and rigidity to the water/HA complex – GAGs, which separate the fibers. HA keeps the fibers from bunching up or aggregating and forming visible aberrations in the vitreous.

HA supplements can substantially improve the tissues inside your eyes, keeping your sight clear and your eyes bright.

Anti-aging fact:
Hyaluronic Acid helps prevent interstitial cystitis incontinence

Hyaluronic Acid gives hope to those who suffer from interstitial cystitis, whose cause is unknown. What is known is the bladder lining has holes in it. This causes the Hyaluronic Acid behind the lining to leak out into the urine, thus causing inflammation, incontinence, and tremendous pain.

Analysis of the urine of interstitial cystitis patients showed HA higher than is found in healthy bodies. Since bladder HA is below the epithelium, this finding may indicate leakage across the epithelium into the urine in interstitial cystitis patients. That knowledge can lead to positive treatment.

Ask your doctor. He surely knows what you now know: Conventional medicine has not overlooked Hyaluronic Acid.

Look at the effectiveness of this compound! HA has been used as a lubricant in eye surgery for over a decade. Dermatologists now inject high-molecular weight HA into the skin to reduce wrinkles. Orthopedists inject HA into the knees, shoulders, sacroiliac, intervertebral discs, and the TM joint to reduce symptoms of osteoarthritis. The success rate of HA in relieving joint problems is about 80%. HA is now being used in prescription eye drops, in skin preparations, and to prevent adhesions following surgery.

The Hyaluronic Acid revolution is under way. How can it help you?

CHAPTER ELEVEN

Lion's Mane

King of the Health-Jungle:
Lion's Mane for Brain Regeneration

What is the relationship between a roaring lion and a small mushroom?

The answer will surprise you if you haven't known about Lion's Mane before. Lion's Mane - technically Hericium erinaceus, and sometimes called Bear's Head or Monkey's Head - is a gourmet mushroom whose texture when cooked has been compared to seafood. The name stems from its cascade of off-white tendrils, somewhat resembling, in miniature, the rich mane of a lion. It often is called "the pom-pon mushroom."

Although relatively new as a valuable supplement elsewhere, Lion's Mane has been a staple in Chinese medicine for hundreds of years. In China, folklore calls it the source of "nerves of steel and the memory of a lion." Only recently have contemporary health food resources recognized the value of Lion's Mane, not only as an anti-oxidant but also as an anti-aging helper.

Documented benefits of Lion's Mane

- Regenerates brain neurons
- Improves cognitive function
- Aides the digestive system
- Kills MRSA
- Helps to prevent Osteoporosis
- Cleans out gastrointestinal toxins

Anti-MRSA – Fighting the scourge of staph infections
Germs often are smarter than we are.

The pesky Methicillin-resistant Staphylococcus aureus - commonly known as MRSA - has developed a nasty resistance to most antibiotics. Got an infection? Chances are very strong that MRSA will work its way into that infection. (Staphylococci bacteria are in the systems of most healthy people, without ever surfacing.)

For those with weakened immune systems and those who are ill from a variety of medical conditions, MRSA is a constant threat.

We'll discuss the "erinacines" in Lion's Mane later in this chapter. Don't let that strange noun scare you. In fact, let that strange noun make you happy, because it's one of the elements in Lion's Mane that enables this substance to fight staph infections.

Turning Lion's Mane loose on osteoporosis

Throughout our lifetimes, our older bones are dissolving as they are replaced by new bone.

But what if hormonal imbalance lets these older bones dissolve … without replacement by new bones? That happens when hormone deficiency accompanies aging.

Lion's Mane comes to the rescue by suppressing the formation of osteoclasts, the villain in our bodies that prevents bone formation. And a superb advantage Lion's Mane has over a number of prescription medications is that it has no cytotoxicity – that is, it doesn't cause any damage to the body's cells.

Reversing the symptoms of Alzheimer's Disease:

Much of the research into the cause and treatment of Alzheimer's Disease has been in Japan. A leading researcher, Dr. Hirozaku Kawagishi of Shizoka University, in 1991 demonstrated the effectiveness of Lion's Mane in stimulating the synthesis of Nerve Growth Factor (NGF), whose lack is regarded as a major cause of Alzheimer's Disease.

Carrying his research further, Dr. Kawagishi showed that brain neurons, destroyed by ongoing Alzheimer's, can be protected by an element in Lion's Mane. So Lion's Mane has two separate and distinct substances with clinically-demonstrated effectiveness in battling damage to the human brain caused by Aklzheimer's.

An associate of Dr. Kawagishi, Dr. Cun Zhuang, now heads product development at Maitake Products, INC. His company has isolated an extract from Lion's Mane that, in an animal study at China Pharmaceutical University, showed even greater anti-Alzheimer's effectiveness than the leading prescription medicine, Aricept.

(In addition to Aricept, a Pfizer product, other FDA-approved Alzheimer's products are Exelon by Novartis, Reminyl by Janssen, and Cognex by First Horizon. All give only temporary relief. All have unfavorable side-effects. None leads to improvement.)

Dr. Cun Zhuang's Lion's Mane extract, in its preliminary studies, showed strong and sometimes dramatic improvement, always with no side-effects whatever.

Stimulating "Nerve Growth Factor"

Lion's Mane came to the attention of researchers who were studying treatments for Alzheimer's disease, looking for compounds that stimulate Nerve Growth Factor (NGF) production in the brain. NGF is part of a family of proteins that play a role in the maintenance, survival and regeneration of neurons during adult life. Its absence in the adult brain of mice leads to a condition resembling Alzheimer's disease.

(The protein molecule NGF was discovered by Rita Levi-Montalcini and isolated by Stanley Cohen, for which they jointly received the 1986 Nobel Prize for Medicine. It is synthesized in minute amounts in all vertebrate tissues.)

A group of Japanese researchers have patented an extraction process, which isolates a Nerve Growth Stimulant Factor – NGSF. They found a compound in Lion's Mane which causes brain neurons to re-grow, a feat of great importance in potentially helping senility, repairing neurological degradation, increasing intelligence and improving reflexes. (Studies also confirm many of its uses, supporting the digestive system, and acting as a tonic for the nervous system. We'll get to those, but first let's explore the way Lion's Mane boosts brain activity.)

Crossing the blood-brain barrier

The problem researchers had to overcome was that Nerve Growth Factor in its original state couldn't be used as an orally administered drug to regenerate brain tissue because it doesn't cross the blood-brain barrier. Ah! they reasoned. If active substances with low molecular weight can be found that do penetrate the barrier and induce the synthesis of NGF inside the brain, such substances then could be taken orally.

And even if these substances can't cross the blood-brain barrier, the enhancement of NGF production would be beneficial for disorders of the marginal nervous system since NGF has a similar effect on neurons in the periphery. This is where the use of the herb Lion's Mane comes into play … and the reason so many refer to Lion's Mane as "The brain tonic."

Paul Stamets, one of the world's leading mycologists and author of a number of authoritative reference works on medical mushrooms, labels the substance this way: "Lion's Mane mushroom mycelium is nature's nutrients for your neurons."

Lion's Mane mushroom contains at least two types of compounds - the hericenones and erinacines - that strongly stimulate NGF synthesis "in vitro" (literally, within the glass, the technique of performing a given experiment in a controlled environment outside of a living organism – for example, in a test tube). Both of these types of substances have the potential to cross the blood-brain barrier. The question has been: Do these substances work when given orally to human patients?

To answer this question, a study was done in a rehabilitative hospital in the Gunma prefecture in Japan, with 50 patients in an experimental group and 50 patients used as a control. All patients were elderly and suffered from cerebrovascular disease, degenerative orthopedic disease, Parkinson's disease, and disabilities stemming from spinal cord injury.

Seven of the patients in the experimental group suffered from various types of dementia. The patients in this group received 5 grams of dried Lion's Mane mushroom per day in their soup for a six-month period. All patients were evaluated before and after the treatment period for their "Functional Independence Measure" (FIM) - the measure of independence in physical capabilities such as eating, dressing, and walking - plus "Perceptual Capacities" - understanding, communication, and memory.

What were the results?

After six months of taking Lion's Mane, six of the seven dementia patients demonstrated improvements in their perceptual capacities, and all seven had improvements in their overall FIM score!

So one of the most exciting areas of the potential of Lion's Mane is its ability to help combat some of the symptoms and underlying causes of dementia and Alzheimer's disease as well as peripheral neurological dysfunction.

The numbers of sufferers needing some type of NGF replacement therapy is soaring by the day, and no cure is in sight from modern medicine. Finally, after all those years in which the curative effects verified by Chinese and Japanese doctors had largely been ignored, a growing number of people are turning to Lion's Mane as a real way to slow down and reverse the symptoms of these devastating diseases. And the effectiveness is not tainted by the possibility of unpleasant side effects. That claim can't be matched by many, if any, of the more painful and more expensive techniques, procedures, and medicines.

Lion's Mane for other ailments

At this writing, no cure exists for HIV and its deadly consequence, AIDS.

But hope exists for relief of the pain associated with HIV, and Lion's Mane can be a major player in that arena. To explain how Lion's Mane can be effective in this difficult circumstance, let's get technical for just a moment:

A substance called erinacine has been shown to increase nerve growth in the central nervous system of rats. Erinacine promotes NGF production throughout the body, and so it helps alleviate the symptoms of peripheral neurological dysfunction. Dr. Will Boggs reported in Neurology magazine that NGF significantly improves the pain symptoms of HIV-infected patients with sensory neuropathy, which affects the sensory nerves - the nerves responsible for sensation throughout the body. Sensory neuropathy most commonly affects the feet, legs, hands, and arms. The symptoms may include numbness or a loss of sensation, coldness, tingling, burning, and extreme sensitivity to touch. And sensory neuropathy affects more than a third of all AIDS patients.

Dr. Giovanni Schifitto from the University of Rochester, New York studied the safety and effectiveness of human NGF for HIV-associated distal sensory neuropathy in 200 affected patients. Their symptoms were significantly alleviated with the administration of the NGF.

As the numbers of sufferers needing some type of NGF replacement therapy climbs ever higher, and with no cure in sight from modern medicine, many people are starting to turn to Lion's Mane as a genuine way to slow down and reverse the symptoms of not only HIV but other devastating diseases whose victims suffer from sensory neuropathy.

Lion's Mane has also been shown to help regulate blood sugar and cholesterol levels. It is completely safe, showing NO signs of toxicity or side effects in any of the major scientific research projects for which it has been the subject. Repeat: Lion's Mane is completely safe, showing NO signs of toxicity or side effects in any of the major scientific research projects for which it has been the subject.

Lion's Mane for better digestion

Unquestionably Lion's Mane has beneficial digestive tonic effects. It is used for treating stomach disorders, duodenal ulcers, and chronic atrophic gastritis, and it improves the discomforts of indigestion.

Clinical studies have shown that ingredients found in Lion's Mane stimulate induction of interferons and modulation of the immune system. How? By boosting the white blood cell count to help the healing process. The powerful substances found in Lion's Mane also enhance the function of the gastric mucus barrier, and the result not only is acceleration of the healing of ulcers, but also anti-inflammatory effects.

And there's even more:

Even aside from its medicinal advantages, Lion's Mane can be a worthwhile – and tasty – addition to the diet.

Gourmet chefs point out that the mushroom in its original form, not as a bottled supplement in powder or tablet form, is unusually delicious. The taste is reminiscent of lobster if Lion's Mane is properly prepared. One source suggests preparing Lion's Mane lightly sautéed in a mixture of olive oil and butter, with just enough heat to turn the tendrils a golden brown.

Aficionados enjoy Lion's Mane in soup, as a substitute for rice, noodles, or pastas. Others add it as a taste-helper in stir-fry.

And in addition:

Lion's Mane also is a source of a substance called beta-glucans. Beta-glucans are often referred to as "biological response modifiers" because they have the ability to activate the immune system.

As is true of every supplement and every prescription medication and every surgical procedure and every generalization relative to human health, exceptions exist. No substance can claim absolute capability, and that situation certainly is true of beta-glucans, especially since so many types of glucans exist.

Still, evidence is impressive.

Chinese doctors regularly prescribe Lion's Mane as a curative for problems of the digestive tract such as stomach and duodenal ulcers, as well as for cancers of the esophagus, stomach and duodenum. This is serious use, well beyond any claims made in the United States. But the efficacy of beta-glucans is accepted everywhere.

Beta-Glucan has been used as an immunoadjuvant therapy for cancer since 1980, primarily in Japan. Numerous studies report that beta-1, 3 glucan has anti-tumor and anti-cancer activity.

The next chunk of technical wording will be significant to those who may have in their family a loved one suffering from a tumor, even a cancerous one:

In a significant study, intralesional administration of beta-1,3 glucans resulted in rapid tumor shrinkage. In another study with mice, beta 1,3 glucan in conjunction with interferon gamma inhibited both the establishment of tumors and liver metastasis.

In some studies, beta-1,3 glucans enhanced the effects of chemotherapy. In studies on bladder cancer with mice, administration of cyclophosphamide, in conjunction with beta-1,3 glucans derived from yeast resulted in reduced mortality. In human patients with advanced gastric or colorectal cancer, the administration of beta-1,3 glucans derived from shiitake mushrooms, in conjunction with chemotherapy resulted in prolonged survival times compared against a control group receiving identical chemotherapy.

Preclinical studies have shown that a soluble yeast beta-glucan product, when used in combination with certain "monoclonal" antibodies or cancer vaccines, offers significant improvements in long-term survival versus monoclonal antibodies alone.

Skeptics exist, of course, but even the most negatively-inclined skeptics agree that Lion's Mane, rich in beta-glucans, has a positive effect on digestion ... and that includes digestive disorders.

We have to conclude that...

Clinical evidence now proves that adding Lion's Mane to the diet can prevent the breakdown in healthy neurological function.

Commercially, Lion's Mane is available in capsule, tablet, or powder form. As a natural aid to better health, no prescription is required.

To repeat a point made earlier: No negative side effects are known to exist. So why don't more people join the trend to add Lion's Mane to their daily diet? Probably because not enough people even know the name Lion's Mane, let alone know the benefits it can offer.

Adding Lion's Mane to the typical person's supplemental requirements would go a long way to improve the quality and length of life. In one long but vital sentence:

The fact that one food source is able to provide the body with the nutrients it needs to stimulate nerve cell regeneration, along with the immune-enhancing properties of beta gleans in healing the digestive tract of ulcers and cancers, is nothing short of remarkable.

CHAPTER TWELVE

Maca

The Maca Root: The Naturally Intelligent Hormone Regulator for Men and Women

Do you or does someone in your household suffer from any of these maladies?

- PMS?
- Erectile dysfunction?
- Low energy and endurance?
- Depression anxiety or stress?
- Poor skin, gums and teeth?
- Peri-menopause, menopause, and post-menopause?
- Memory loss?
- Infertility?

Quite possibly, the debilitating culprit is an imbalance to your Endocrine System (our internal hormone regulator).

Here's what happens when the equilibrium of our hormones gets churned up: Our entire internal eco-system goes into overdrive and our wires get crossed – much like a computer that's caught a destructive bug – destroying its own internal drive so fast we can't effect a repair quickly enough or hard enough to save it.

The good news and the bad news

The bad news first: Unfortunately, the most commonly prescribed for hormone imbalance is Hormone Replacement Therapy (HRT). But even natural hormone replacement therapy can cause what we've just described. It's no surprise that Western medicine works on the symptoms of these problems rather than the whole "ball of wax." I'm sure you'll agree that it's time to look at what's actually causing our symptoms to occur and find ways to regulate the Endocrine System as a whole.

Fortunately, we still can turn to Nature for the answer. Within the bounty of Nature exists a foolproof medicinal therapy that keeps our Endocrine System (our internal hormone regulator) healthy by 100-fold: The Maca Root. Its unique qualities work on the entire Endocrine System rather than merely replacing hormones piecemeal, the way modern medicine does.

The super-natural benefits of the Maca Root

Maca Root works wonders in a huge number of ways. It gives you:

- Increased energy and endurance.
- Greater stamina.
- Stronger sexual prowess.
- Increased fertility.
- Better hormonal regulation.
- Alleviates depression, anxiety and stress.
- Improved circulatory system.
- Improved memory, learning, and mental acuity.
- A more radiant appearance for your skin.
- Help in fighting off anemia, rickets, osteomalacia, and stomach cancer.
- Healthy teeth and gums.
- Powerful anti-fungi and anti-bacteria agent.

The juice that keeps our moods stable, metabolism stable, and reproductive systems and sexual enjoyment from depleting.

Maca History: The Incans found Maca Root so potent in its rich super-food and medicinal properties; they restricted its use to Royal families. It was later, in the 1600s that Spaniards recorded its medicinal properties, confirming what the native healers of the Andes already knew. In the 1960s and later in the 1980s, German and North American scientists analyzed its nutritional properties and rekindled the interest in the Maca Root and designated it as the "lost crops of the Andes."

The foundation of the endocrine system is the network of glands and the hormones they produce. The glands of our regulatory system release over 20 major hormones directly into our bloodstream and influence almost every cell, organ, and function of our bodies. These chemical messengers transfer information and instructions from one set of cells to another. Each hormone affects only the cells genetically programmed to receive and respond to its message. Hormone levels can be influenced by factors such as stress, infection, and changes in the balance of fluid and minerals in the blood.

Especially as we age, our hormones have a tendency to deplete, or change -- and our bodies begin to malfunction. It only makes sense that in order to stop premature aging; we need to regulate and sometimes quick-start our hormones into producing as a unified system.

Maca Root's regulating properties

The Maca Root is a rare member of the radish family (found only in the upper regions of the Andes Mountains in Peru). This magical root contains a storehouse of medicinal properties rich with amino acids, vitamins, minerals, sterols, fatty acids, glucosinates, and the recently discovered alkaloids (tannins and saponins). It has more than 55 naturally-occurring, beneficial phyto-chemicals. These naturally-occurring chemicals include important hormonal precursors and sterols that have been proved time and time again to assist the human body in a number of recognizable ways. Most people feel their mood and energy level lift in an instant.

Important Note: Too much or too little of any hormone is harmful to your body

Here's the difference between HRT and Maca Root: Maca Root does not contain any hormones. Rather, its action on the body jogs the pituitary gland into producing the precursor hormones that ultimately wind up raising estrogen, progesterone, and testosterone levels, when and where they're needed. They balance the adrenal glands, the thyroid, and the pancreas. Finding a way to keep the Endocrine System communicating should be the therapeutic choice … rather than throwing the entire body into a dangerous state of confusion with time-bomb drugs.

Men as well as women need hormone balancing

Let's face it - the old adage is that women usually have frightening hormonal episodes. You've heard it said often enough. "Her hormones must be off…" or "She must be going through menopause…" Although there's a lot of press about women needing hormonal therapy, we all need it -- especially as we age. Yes, men need stabilizing too.

The benefits for men are:
- Increased energy,
- More stamina,
- Higher athletic performance,
- Heightened virility and fertility rate,
- Eliminated problems of erectile dysfunction,
- Hormonal Balance,
- Increased testosterone levels.

The benefits for women are:
- Relief of peri/post and menopausal symptoms,
- Zero hot flashes,
- Hormonal balance,
- Increased fertility,
- Improved sexual stimulation,
- Increased energy,
- New-found stamina,
- Greater athletic performance,
- Fewer PMS symptoms.

The medicinal and nutritious alternative to hormone balancing is the life-enhancing discovery everyone should be grateful for

The scientist most responsible for our knowledge of the Maca Root is Dr. Gloria Chacon, a trained biologist at the University of San Marcos, in Lima, Peru.

Maca Root works totally different from HRT. Instead of replacing hormones, Maca Root assists the hypothalamus and the pituitary to work at optimal capacity, which in turn improves the work of all the endocrine glands. The implications of Dr. Chacon's work on the pituitary effects of the Maca Root are enormous.

Dr. Chacon's discovery implies that Hormone Replacement Therapy (HRT) will no longer be the gold standard for improving our health -- even from a holistic viewpoint.

The undisputed effects of hormone balancing

Dr. Chacon later went on to isolate four alkaloids from the Maca Root. She gave female and male rats either powdered Maca Root or the four alkaloids (tannins and saponins) isolated from the roots of the Maca.

Her famous experiment with female and male rats changed the way we look at hormone balancing. She had a group of mice that weren't given either Maca Root or the alkaloids from the Maca Root. Another group received Maca Root powder. Yet another group was given the alkaloids from the Maca Root. When she compared the control groups, she found that those that received either the Maca Root or the alkaloids from the root showed multiple egg follicles in the females, while the males had a much higher sperm count than the other group that hadn't been given the supplements.

Dr. Chacon established clearly that it was the alkaloids in the Maca Root that produced fertility effects on the ovaries and testes of the rats and, not its plant hormones. The effects could be measured, too, in as little as seven hours.

She concluded that the alkaloids acted on the hypothalamus and pituitary glands. This tells us: Not only does Maca Root have an effect on the ovaries and testes but also on the adrenals, pancreas and thyroid as well showing positive effects on hormonal balancing issues such as hot flashes, memory problems, fatigue, mood swings, and male impotence. The implications of Chacon's discovery of the pituitary stimulating effects of Maca are, to say the least, astounding.

The bad, the ugly and the horror of Hormone Replacement Therapy

Based on the important research of Dr. Chacon, more and more doctors are using Maca Root instead of Hormone Replacement Therapy. Of course, HRT has been the medical field's answer to hormonal imbalances for years. I think a better word for HRT should be hormone deregulation. HRT is shown to shut down the glands that naturally produce hormones.

You may say, "That doesn't make sense." But take look at this:
Dr. Jorge Malaspina, respected cardiologist, explains: "Replacement hormones circulating in the endocrine system send a message to the pituitary gland and the hypothalamus that they've already produced a sufficient quantity of hormones in the body. You can imagine what happens next - they stop producing hormones altogether. Or look at it this way - the pituitary gland shuts down." When our hormones become imbalanced, havoc breaks loose on our system. If our Endocrine System starts failing, we can suffer from depression, our sexual drive goes down the tubes, and we experience drastic skin changes, weakness, fatigue, obesity, diabetes, decreased hormonal levels, hyperthyroidism, and hypothyroidism and menopausal dysfunctions.

Dr. Malaspina goes on to say: "When menopause arrives, the ovaries are atrophied and don't produce the estrogen and progesterone which the body requires to function." For this reason, he states: "I encourage women to start using Maca before menopause. It seems to help the endocrine system to stay in balance."

Maca keeps your hormones balanced and your age a secret

American Physician Gabriel Cousens, an internist from Patagonia, Arizona, is a wholehearted believer that the Maca Root is the key to counteract the effects of aging on the endocrine system.

Here's why:

Dr. Cousens states that, "Whenever possible, I prefer to use Maca Therapy rather than Hormone Replacement Therapy. HRT has actually been shown to age the body by diminishing the hormone producing capability of the glands." He goes on the say that: "Maca has proved to be extremely effective with menopausal patients as well, by eliminating hot flashes, depression, and giving the patient higher energy levels."

For men: Maca counteracts difficulties with erectile dysfunction they may experience as they age.

Your answer to sexual enhancement

An added bonus for all of us: Maca is truly a sex-enhancing food. The alkaloids in Maca work on the hypothalamus-pituitary axis. Science has now shown us what the Peruvians have known for centuries: the glucosinates and amino acid L-arginine found in Maca stimulate sexual desire in both men and women. For men, it holds incredible curative powers for relieving erectile dysfunction and reviving sexual abilities and stamina (making a 60-year old feel like a teenager again); and for women - well, of course, it eases hormone irregularities, adds much-needed moisture, and muscle tone, besides which, it bestows a huge calming effect.

Maca as an adjunct to whole health treatments

Another example is Dr. Harold Clark's work in New Rochelle, New York. Dr. Clark uses a number of natural therapies such as chelation therapy and ozone therapy in addition to herbs, vitamins, and minerals in his practice. But he was absolutely amazed by how fast Maca root worked, specifically, on two of his patients.

One 55-year-old postmenopausal woman had numerous health problems, including elevated blood sugar levels, hypertension, atrial fibrillation, and low magnesium levels. She'd been ill for two months with osteomyelitis (an infection of the bone), usually caused by microbial agents. Unable to work, she was suffering from great fatigue and depression and feeling worse and worse over the last five years. Within four days of taking the Maca powder, she went through an enormous turnaround. She's gone out to shop in the stores, she's cleaning her house, and she feels strong and vital and part of the human race again.

Most women find that Maca Root is on an entirely different level when it comes to its effectiveness. They've found that phytoestrogen herbs like black cohosh and licorice roots are not on pare with Maca Root.

Maca's fight against anemia, menopause, impotence, sterility premature aging, weakness and chronic fatigue

Dr. Jorge Calderon, Internist and former Chief of the Department of Biological Sciences and Dean of the Faculty of Human Medicine at the National

> *Footnote for men: Because the endocrine glands slow down when we age, men begin to experience difficulty in maintaining good sexual relationships. Not to worry – move over, Viagra - Maca reverses these effects in no time.*

University of Federico Villarreal in Lima, Peru, is a pioneer in the therapeutic applications of the Maca Root. He's found that Maca, along with prescribing an excellent diet and certain lifestyle changes, helps male impotency, male and female sterility, and chronic fatigue. Besides the traditional uses for Maca Root, he's found that Maca's curative properties treat rickets, anemia, osteoporosis, and bone fractures.

Beware – HRT might be dangerous for women with breast implants

Dr. Hugo Malaspina, a well-respected cardiologist, found that Maca was the treatment of choice for women who have had breast augmentation. A case in point: His 49-year old patient had a hysterectomy 9 years prior. Although she still had her ovaries, she began to have menopausal symptoms. Because she had breast implants, the usual hormone replacement therapy wasn't an option. He started her on Maca Root and within three months the depression, constipation, and hot flashes cleared up completely.

Early onset menopause due to hysterectomies

This deserves special note because there are over one million women in the U.S. alone who have undergone complete hysterectomies who no longer have their ovaries.

In a recent interview Dr. Malaspina was cited as saying: "Because so many women have had their ovaries taken out – they're told that hormone replacement therapy is a necessity (which only benefits the pharmaceutical companies). Not true: Women who have had hysterectomies – and rapidly. The Maca Root should be mentioned as one of the best and danger-free supplements for the symptoms of early onset menopause."

Help for sufferers of Hyperthyroidism and Hypothyroidism

Another huge accolade for Maca is the effect it has on balancing our adrenals. Dr. Henry Campanile offers adrenal balancing therapy in his practice. His therapy is based around the medicinal properties of the Maca Root because of its balancing and nourishing effects on the adrenal glands. Maca is an extremely rich source for its minerals and iodine, which is vital for the regulating the Endocrine System due to its effect on balancing the thyroid gland.

Give the control back to Nature

It's conclusive – we all grow old. The ups and downs of our hormones are a vicious cycle, and a part of growing older. Unfortunately for us, our Western culture believes we can improve what nature so bounteously provides us. Our food sources have been destroyed, with hydroponics, sugars, additives, chemicals, preservatives, and hormones we put in our bodies every day.

Because of this, the reality is we need additional help to get our glands working again. By supplementing with the most natural form of hormone balancing, we can keep these imbalances from sending our bodies into a state of confusion.

Nature's limitless ability to renew us with this of medicinal and nutritional plant is frankly awe-inspiring.

How much should you take? Personally, I've been taking 12,000mg every day, so I use the powdered Maca. Not only have I found that the Maca Root gives me so much more energy, but my hormonal health has improved tremendously.

No known side effects exist. The most evident of this statement: hundreds of years of consumption in Peru.

CHAPTER THIRTEEN

Maqui Berry

Maqui Berry:
Arm Yourself Against Age-related Diseases

Today, we hear a lot of "hype" about the importance of supplementing our diets with fruits rich in antioxidants.

Scientists and researchers are finding that the power of natural nutrients in fruits and vegetables help combat a number of aging diseases. And the USDA, American Heart Association, American Cancer Society, National Academy of Sciences and American Diabetes Association all urge Americans to eat more fruits and vegetables every day.

How much fruits and vegetables do we need to consume?
Nutritionists recommend we consume at least 5 servings of fruits and vegetables per day to see a huge decrease in heart disease, cancer, high blood pressure and more. Add 2 more additional portions of fruits and vegetables a day and you'll see an 11% increase in your functional health..

On the average, American don't get the minimum 5 servings of fruits and vegetables needed to stay healthy- let alone an extra 2 portions. The outcome? We're slowly poisoning ourselves with processed foods, filled with refined sugars and fillers - all in the name of convenience. Due to the prevalent onslaught of disease we're getting one wake-up call we can't ignore: We need to drastically increase our antioxidant intake to nourish our bodies and fight disease.

I know it's difficult for most of us to start the healthy habit of eating at least 5 to 15 different organic fruits and vegetables on a daily basis. We may not have the time to shop, cook, or even find time to eat them all!

So here's a good solution: Supplementing our diets with high antioxidant superfruits can reduce the amount of servings we need to eat for a healthy aging process.

A new wave of exotic fruits is surfacing on the market today. Acai, pomegranate, goji berry, noni, mangosteen, seaberry, and the familiar blueberry, cranberry, and red grape are major players in the new class of fruits called Superfruits. Aptly named for their myriad of nutrients, including vitamins, minerals, carotenoids, phytosterols, essential acids, and amino acids, all of which play a major role to promote health and prevent disease. These antioxidants help support a healthy immune response, aid digestion, maintain healthy heart function, support healthy blood sugar levels, promote healthy joint function, and even help protect our bodies from free radicals which is a key factor in healthy aging. These Superfruits are recognized antioxidant sources, along with the research to back up their claims.

The new Superfruit: Maqui Berry

Maqui is a deep colored purple berry collected from the distant Patagonia region which stretches from central Chile to Antarctica, and considered one of the cleanest places on this planet. The Mapuche Indians have traditionally used the berry for centuries for its powerful medicinal properties that help them with a variety of ailments such as sore throat, diarrhea, ulcers, hemorrhoids, birth delivery, fever, tumors and other ailments.

The Mapuche Indians are the only Indians in South America that weren't conquered by any European countries. According to a 16th century document written by the Spaniards, the Mapuche warriors drank a fermented beverage call "chicha" made from maqui berry several times daily. This practice may have contributed to the warriors extraordinary strength and stamina.

Aging & Free Radicals

As we age, our cells are increasingly affected by nasty free radicals. Our organs begin to degenerate and the aging process speeds up. Free radicals are unstable, destructive molecules, created as a natural biological process by the body. They emerge from almost anything our bodies do that involves oxygen. This includes digestive functions and breathing. The good news is that our bodies are naturally equipped with built-in defense mechanisms to protect themselves from free radical damage. The bad news is that these defense mechanisms begin to deteriorate as we age, leaving our bodies almost incapable of keeping free radicals at bay.

Science has long held that damage by oxygen free radicals is behind many of the maladies that come with aging, including cardiovascular disease and cancer. There's firm evidence that a high intake of fruits and vegetables reduces risk of cancer, where a low intake raises the risk. Recent evidence suggests that diminished brain function associated with aging and disorders such as Alzheimer's and Parkinson's diseases may be due to increased vulnerability to free radicals.

Antioxidants

Antioxidants contain an extra oxygen molecule that neutralize free radicals before they do any harm. Our bodies produce natural antioxidants to combat oxidative stress and inflammation.

However, the aging process and the various environmental and life-style stressors such as smoking, pollution, sun radiation, chemicals in the food, all create more free radicals than our bodies can naturally fight off. Maqui berry is jam-packed with antioxidants, especially the anthocyanins and polyphenols, to help neutralize the free radicals and reduce oxidative stress.

Comparing & Measuring Antioxidants

Many methods exist to measure antioxidant level. One of the most common methods is call ORAC, which was developed by food nutrition researchers at Tufts University. The ORAC test measures a food's antioxidant ability to neutralize free radicals and potentially mitigate health imbalances.

Nutritionists recommend at least 5 servings of fruits and vegetables daily, which is around 2500 ORAC per day. For optimal health, we should consume 12,000 ORAC daily. Most Americans don't ever consume the minimum 2500 ORAC units recommended.

Comparing the Maqui Berry to other fruits, it seems the Maqui Berry contains one of the highest ORAC value of any other known fruits. It contains 34 times higher ORAC value than bananas, 22 times higher value than red grapes, 8 times higher value than strawberries, 6 times higher value than raspberries, 4 times higher value than blueberries, and almost 3 times higher value than pomegranates.

Take a look at the chart below measuring the ORAC content of the different types of fruits:

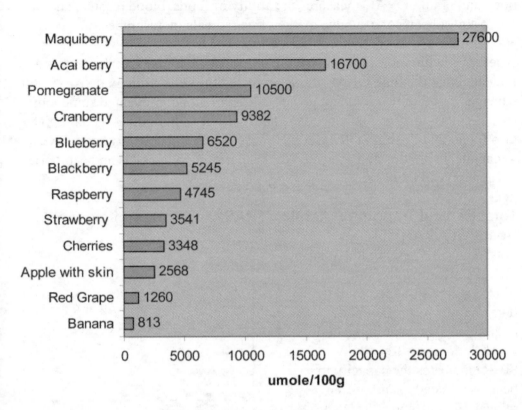

ORAC value of various fruits per 100g serving

When comparing spray dried powder, maqui spray dried powder is 3 times higher than acai spray dried powder; and maqui fruit & seed powder is almost 3 times higher than acai fruit & skin freezed dried powder.

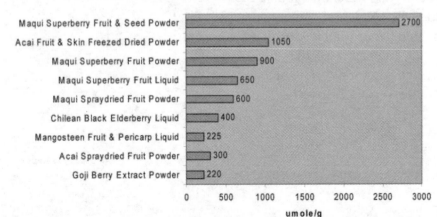

ORAC Value of Various Fruit Powder & Liquid per1 gram Serving

High ORAC Fruits May Stall Aging and Aid Memory

Studies conducted at the Jean Mayer USDA Human Nutrition Research Center on Aging at Tufts University in Boston, suggest that consuming fruits and vegetables with a high-ORAC value may help slow the aging process in both body and brain. ORAC measures the ability of foods, blood plasma, and just about any substance to subdue oxygen free radicals in test tubes.

After testing the ingestion of High ORAC foods in animals, early evidence indicated that the high ORAC foods protected the cells from oxidative damage, raised the antioxidant power in human blood, prevented some long-term memory loss, and enhanced the ability to learn in middle-aged rats. They also found that the high ORAC foods caused the brain cells to respond well to chemical stimulus and protected the rats' tiny blood vessels and capillaries against oxygen damage.

Total Radical Trapping Potential (TRAP) and Total Antioxidant Reactivity (TAR)

Total Radical Trapping Potential (TRAP) measures the amount of free radicals trapped in the body and the total amount of antioxidants present in the body. Total Antioxidant Reactivity (TAR) indicates the capacity to decrease a steady state of free radical concentration. Total phenols is positively correlate to TRAP and TAR. According to a research published in Journal of Agricultural & Food Chemistry, Maqui berry contains much higher polyphenol content and scored better for TRAP and TAR when compared to red wine, blackberry, strawberry, blueberry, cranberry, and raspberry.

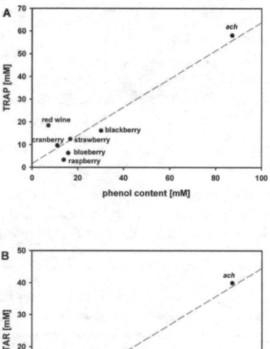

TEAC, ORAC, FRAP, DPPH Antioxidant Measurement

Because no single antioxidant assay can accurately reflect the antioxidant potency of any beverage, we used four tests to measure antioxidant potency:

1. Trolox equivalent antioxidant capacity (TEAC)
2. Oxygen radical absorbing capacity (ORAC)
3. Ferric reducing antioxidant power (FRAP)
4. Free radical scavenging properties by the diphenyl-1-picrylhydrazyl (DPPH) radical

	DPPH (% Inhibited)	ORAC (umole of TE/ml)	FRAP (umole of FE/ml)	TEAC (umole/ml)
Maqui Berry Juice	207.7	133	55.0	127.8
Pomegranate Juice	50.1	25	8.1	41.6
Red Wine	35.2	25.7	4.3	18.7
Blueberry Juice	20.6	20.6	4.2	15.0
Cranberry Juice	19.2	15.4	2.7	10.4
Acai Juice	18.3	19.5	3.8	12.8
Orange Juice	12.7	7.4	1.5	4.2
Apple Juice	11.8	4.8	1.2	3.6

Anthocyanins - The most powerful Antioxidant compound

Anthocyanins are antioxidant flavonoids that protect many of the body's systems and contain the strongest physiological effects of any plant compounds. One study found, Anthocyanins to have the strongest antioxidizing power of 150 flavonoids. (Approximately 4,000 different flavonoids have been identified.)

Anthocyanins are produced by plants for self-protection against, sun, irradiation, diseases, and biological enemies. The harsh cold weather and the high solar radiation in Central and Southern Chile guarantee high anthocyanins in the fruits and berries, including the Maqui Berries that are grown in that region.

Studies show that anthocyanins have a profoundly positive influence on a variety of health conditions. One reason is their anti-inflammatory properties, which affect collagen and

	Anthocyanins (mg/100g)
Red Wine	24-35
Red Grape	30-750
Boysenberry	160
Cherry	350-400
Blackberry	82-325 (mostly 150)
Cranberry	50-80
Red Raspberry	213-428
Blueberry	25-495
Bilberry	300-648
Mangosteen Powder	195
Acai Powder	320
Maqui Berry Powder	**4000-5000**

the nervous system. Their ability to protect both large and small blood vessels from oxidative damage derives from a range of effects, including mitigating microvessel damage from high blood-sugar levels that cause complications in diabetes 2.

In an animal study conducted by a group of Bulgarian researchers, the test group was given a compound of histamine and serotonin, both of which cause allergic reactions and increase capillary permeability. Later the animals were supplemented with flavonoids. The Anthocyanins showed an anti-inflammatory ability and dampened the allergic reactions.

Another animal study illustrates how cyanidins, found in most fruit sources of anthocyanins, functioned as a potent antioxidant, protected cell membrane lipids from oxidation by a variety of harmful substances, and is four times more powerful an antioxidant than vitamin E.

Maqui Berry contains one of the highest anthocyanin levels compared to many fruits and vegetables; more than 100 times more than a glass of red wine, and more than 10 times the level of acai spray dried powder. Take a look at the chart below.

Maqui berries contain very high amounts of anthocyanins, (purple phenols with powerful antioxidant properties) which were found to demonstrate many potential therapeutic effects including lowering of oxidized LDL cholesterol levels and help combat premature aging. The primary anthocyanin in Maqui berries is delpinidin 3-sambucosies-5-glucoside.

Maqui Berry Lowers Inhibition of Human LDL Oxidation

Cholesterol is not inherently harmful. It actually serves many essential purposes in our bodies. For instance, it acts as the main precursor for testosterone and estrogen. However, it is well known that alterations in cholesterol levels and ratios, (i.e, increased total cholesterol, low high-density lipoprotein (HDL) cholesterol, and elevated low-density lipoprotein (LDL) cholesterol) are proven risk factors for heart disease. LDL must be protected against damage from free radicals - the process that creates oxidized LDL.

Thisoxidized, or damaged form of LDL that research has identified as an important factor in initiating atherosclerosis. Oxidized LDL cholesterol causes impairment of endothelial cell function in artery walls, inhibition of nitric oxide production by blood vessel cells, enhancement of the release of inflammatory cytokines, and increased the ability of white blood cells to stick to and traverse artery walls.

According to a research published in Journal of Agricultural & Food Chemistry, Maqui berry effectively inhibits copper induced LDL oxidation. In human endothelial cell cultures, Maqui berry significantly protects the body from hydrogen peroxide induced intracellular oxidative stress.

The French Paradox and Polyphenols
According to FAO data (a world-wide quality monitoring system), the average French person consumed 108 grams per day of fat from animal sources in 2002, while the average American consumed only 72. The French eat four times more butter, 60 percent more cheese, and nearly three times more pork. Although the French consume only slightly more total fat (171 g/d vs. 157), they consume much more saturated fat. However, according to data from the British Heart foundation, in 1999, rates of death from coronary heart disease among males aged 35-74 years were 230 per 100,000 people in the US but only 83 per 100,000 in France.

This discrepancy is labeled the French Paradox. It has been suggested that France's high red wine consumption is a primary factor in the trend. It was initially believed that resveratrol in red wine could be a contributing factor to the French Paradox. Today, researchers believe that it is the polyphenols that may be responsible for the very low incidence of heart disease as the resveratrol concentration in wine seems too low to account for the cardiovascular health benefits. These antioxidant compounds inhibit the oxidation of LDL cholesterol and inhibit the formation of blood clots. The anthocyanins in red wine also protect against coronary heart disease, since these red pigments inhibit cholesterol synthesis. While red wine has a good quantity of polyphenols, Maqui berry has twice as many phenols compared to pomegranate juice and red wine, and 4 times more than acai juice.

Support Healthy Inflammation Response by Reducing NFkappaB
Scientists have discovered many antioxidant-rich fruits can safely, powerfully,

	Phenols (mg/ml)
Maqui Berry Juice	8.36
Pomegranate Juice	3.8
Red Wine	3.5
Blueberry Juice	2.3
Acai Juice	2.1
Cranberry Juice	1.7
Orange Juice	0.7
Apple Juice	0.4

and naturally modulate inflammation. Recent studies have tied inflammation to the over expression of a protein molecule called nuclear factor-kappa beta (NFkB), a key regulator of our immune and inflammatory response system that controls a range of pro-inflammatory cytokines which cause inflammation and pain. NFkB acts like a switch, turning on genes that produce the body's inflammatory responses. Because NFkB's expression increases in aging adults, scientists have sought ways to modulate NFkB and its effects in the body.

Dr Juan Hancke, the chief research scientist from University of Chile, and head scientist for CTI Consortium, a non-profit organization, has recently obtained research funding from World Bank to conduct research on Maqui berry. Since Maqui berry has been traditionally used by the Mapuche Indians to treat sore throat, ulcers, birth delivery, and fever, Dr. Hancke had his team focus on anti-inflammatory research to verify these traditional claims. In vitro research by the team of scientists found that Maqui berry exerted powerful anti-inflammatory effects by inhibiting the over expression of NFkB, thereby reducing cytokines and enzymes that cause inflammation. Various concentrations of Maqui berry reduce the activity of NFkappaB, which is the key regulator of our inflammatory response system.

Activating PPAR gamma

Researchers show us that the activation of PPAR gamma leading to the inhibition of NFkappaB is possible via the activation of PPAR gamma gene. When PPAR gamma is activated, NFkappaB is inhibited, resulting in the reduction of COX-2 enzyme and prostaglandin levels. These pro-inflammatory cytokines cause inflammation and pain in the body. In vitro cell study conducted at the University of Chile showed Maqui berry to activate PPARgamma.

Maqui berry reduces COX-2 Enzymes

In addition to being a potent antioxidant, Dr. Juan Hancke explains that Maqui Berry is a powerful natural COX-2 inhibitor. COX-2 is the enzyme responsible for inflammation and pain. Prostaglandins whose synthesis involves the COX-2 enzyme cause inflammation and pain as well. A team of researchers from University of Rochester Medical Center show that selectively blocking COX-2 enzyme would be beneficial in treating inflammation related diseases. Various groups of researchers also found links between COX-2 and cancer, Alzheimer, arthritis, and other ailments. Scientists now confirm that COX-2 enzyme is triggered by inflammatory cytokines and NFkappaB.

Over expression of COX-2 is related to the development of certain cancers and chronic inflammatory diseases such as arthritis. In vitro research by Dr.

Juan Hancke shows Maqui berry concentrate reduces COX-2 enzyme and acts as a natural way to manage non-chronic inflammation. This is truly a scientific breakthrough in healthy inflammation response. Maqui works with your body's natural chemistry to promote healthy joint function, by targeting multiple enzymes, or pathways.

Maqui berry Destroys Cancer Cells in Lab

Over expression of NF-KB releases potent pro-inflammatory cytokines fostering the growth of tumors. The inhibition of NF-kB can generate apoptosis in cancer cell lines. Several studies by researchers across the country demonstrate the link between COX-2 inhibitors and cancer. These researchers find the use of COX-2 inhibitor to reduce the incidence of colon cancer - and deaths from the disease - by nearly half.

Maqui berry is also used by the Mapuche Indians to treat cancer & ulcer. Dr. Juan Hancke & his scientific team from the University of Chile conducted cancer research with Maqui berry concentrate on CACO2 (human colon cancer cells) to verify its anti-cancer activity. In a human leukemia (HL-60) cell study, different concentrations of Maqui Berry reduced the viability of the HL-60 cells in a 24 hours incubation period and induced cancer cell apoptosis (cell death).

At $30\mu g/\mu l$ concentration of Maqui Berry concentrate, Dr. Hancke's team shows Maqui Berry to be highly effective in eliminating 100% of human colon cancer cells in the petri dish. Please note: This is only a cell-culture model and is not intended to show that Maqui Berry can prevent or treat cancer in people. Experts today are uncertain how much effect antioxidants have on cancer cells in the human body. The factors such as nutrient absorption, metabolism, and the influence of other biochemical processes may influence the antioxidants' chemical activity. Researchers are very encouraged by the findings as compounds that show good activity against cancer cells in a model system and are most likely to have beneficial effects in our bodies.

Organic and Sustainable Harvest Practices

Today, most conventional fruits and vegetables are awash in chemicals, synthetic fertilizers, pesticides, fungicides, and herbicides. These contaminants sneak into our bodies and wreak havoc to our health. Eating organic ingredients is better for our health because it's natural and pure. Organically grown ingredients are also better for the environment, and will help protect our world for future generations.

The Maqui Berries are harvested in the wild, hand-picked by the Mapuche

Indians in a pollution free, pesticide free, certified organic native forest. Using sustainable harvest practice, the Mapuche Indians employ a pruning technique by breaking a soft part of the branch. This increases oxygen absorption for the branches. The leaves and stems are then placed under the tree so they decompose and become a natural fertilizer for the tree. This system prevents trees form getting cut down.

In conclusion:

If you're like most Americans, and you don't consume enough fruits and vegetables to get your sufficient daily recommended antioxidants, try supplementing your diet with the highest, new generation of Superfruit. This superfruit is now available in the United States. Maqui Berry is naturally pure, organic, and clinically tested to help support healthy inflammatory responses, healthy cardiovascular functions, stall premature aging, and help combat many age-related diseases.

CHAPTER FOURTEEN

Monolaurin

The Mothers Have It:
Monolaurin - Master Immune Booster

When bacteriologist Alexander Fleming discovered Penicillin in 1928, a sigh of relief was heard around the globe.

Today, once again, the alarms are sounding … from terror not joy. Stop to think for a minute that in an age in which modern medicine seems limitless, we've landed ourselves right back in the Middle Ages where pestilence, bacterial infections, and viruses were the #1 prime killers.

Got the sniffles? Scratchy throat? These symptoms may not be that easy to get rid of today. At least 20,000 people die every year from the flu. Look around you: It's quite common these days that you or someone you know suffers from a debilitating bacterial or viral infection.

The irony: New strains of bacteria have multiplied with increased strength, and what's worse is that they're often times completely resistant to our antibiotics, leaving our immune system in danger of breaking down completely.

We're fast becoming immune to the effects of antibiotics. The resistance is cumulative, and builds until we're defenseless to fight new strains of viruses and bacterial diseases.

It's true; you may reason that you're safe because you rarely take antibiotics. Oh, but you do. We ingest it in surprising amounts -- without even a thought -- in our food sources every day. The meats we eat are full of antibiotics because the animals are treated with these drugs for therapeutic, disease prevention, and production reasons. And those treatments in turn cause the microbes in our bodies to become resistant to treatment, making human diseases harder to treat.

And it's not only bacteria that develop antibiotic resistance. Viruses develop resistance as well.

You can see the downhill spiral. Safe and effective antiviral remedies are paramount to our safety. Limited antiviral treatments exist in conventional medicine against the vast majority of viruses.

For these reasons, we need to move fast and fight harder, to remedy the situation – especially when new viruses are running rampant and spinning into stronger and deadlier diseases against which our immune systems have no defense.

Monolaurin: The nonresistant all-natural super-immune booster

Don't sound the alarms yet. A new super-immune booster called Monolaurin has been making headlines. Monolaurin is a "monoester" derived from monoglyceride of lauric acid and has profound anti-viral and anti-bacterial effects.

For clarity: "mono" means "one." And an ester is an organic compound formed by the reaction between an alcohol and an acid, with the elimination of water.

Monolaurin is based on lauric acid, first discovered as the main antiviral and antibacterial substance in human breast milk. Lauric acid is a saturated fatty acid also found in coconut products. It's naturally abundant in a mother's milk.

Think about it: From the time we were conceived we were totally dependent on nutrients from our mother's body for our own immune protection. After studying the composition of the mother's milk, medical researchers found a common denominator: high concentrations of monoglyceride lauric acid. This finding is what led researchers to study Monolaurin as a potent anti-viral agent. Its anti-viral power is highly unusual in that it contains properties toxic to lower bacteria, fungi, yeast, and viruses – but yet it's non-toxic to man.

Infectious note: Some organisms are so resistant to **ALL** approved antibiotics so as a last ditch effort they're often times treated with experimental and potentially toxic drugs.

Scientist discovers superconductor for our immune system

Dr. Jon Kabara is popular among his colleagues for discovering the insightful effects of certain lipids (or fatty acids) and their derivatives (one being Monolaurin) to kill bacteria, yeast, fungi, and enveloped viruses. The properties that determined the anti-infective actions of these lipids were related to their structure of free fatty acids and monoglycerides (Monlaurin). The monoglycerides are active; diglycerides and triglycerides are inactive. But of all the saturated fatty acids, the monoglycerides have the greatest antiviral activity shown to kill literally thousands of bacterial strains.

For starters, Dr. Kabara's research has led to some definitive conclusions regarding Monolaurin:

Monolaurin is more biologically active than lauric acid, showing positive results against influenza virus, pneumovirus, paramyxovirus (known as Newcastle), morbillivirus (known as rubeola), coronavirus (avian infectious, bronchitis virus), herpes simplex I & II, CMV, EBV, and HIV. It seems to work this way: Monolaurin disrupts the "lipid bilayer" of the virus, thus preventing the capability of a virus to attach itself to otherwise susceptible host cells. It actually binds to the lipid-protein envelope of the virus, inactivating the virus.

So Monolaurin restrains the replication of viruses by interrupting the binding of virus to host cells and prevents the uncoating of viruses necessary for replication and infection. Dr. Kabara and those who have followed his investigations have shown that Monolaurin can remove all measurable infectivity by directly disintegrating the viral envelope. In one sentence that doesn't require a medical or technical background: Monolaurin, binding itself to the viral envelope, makes a virus more susceptible to host defenses.

Dr. Jon Kabara's findings confirmed

All this makes good theory. But do the researchers have any validation from a major credible source?

They certainly do. The Centers for Disease Control in Atlanta, Georgia conducted their own study focused on Monlaurin-tested strains of viruses. They realized that all the viruses had their own lipid membrane surrounding them. The presence of a lipid membrane on viruses makes them especially vulnerable to Monolaurin. They found that Monolaurin shut down toxic effects enveloped in the cell membranes of 14 human RNA and DNA viruses. Including: flu virus, Herpes Simplex types 1 and 2, Epstein-Barr Virus, Rubella, and cytomegalovirus. Data from these studies suggest that the viruses' loss of infectivity is associated with Monolaurin entering into the virus. Case proved.

Monolaurin's trick:

Monolaurin works its magic by disintegrating the virus' fatty membrane coat. The unassailable data from these studies suggest Monolaurin actually makes its way inside the virus and kills its power for infection.

Now here's the trick: Once Monolaurin enters the virus, the virus in turn begins to absorb the fatty acids so they can begin the replication process. The virus is fooled into literally destroying its own protective envelope. Monolaurin is not only one of the most unusual anti-virals; it also is an effective masquerader. The result is that a virus literally implodes.

That's right. Monolaurin dowses the lipids in fluids within the envelope of the virus, causing the virus to turn on itself and disintegrate its membrane. Conclusion: The fatty acids and monoglycerides attack the enveloped viruses and make them danger-proof, confirming that Kabara's original studies are valid.

Practical uses for Monolaurin

From all this technical jargon you might conclude that Monolaurin is available only by prescription and that probably it has to be administered by injection.

If that were the case, you wouldn't be reading about it here. Monolaurin is available in over-the-counter caplets, usually of 500 milligrams.

The availability itself speaks volumes, because obviously government restrictions would apply if it weren't safe. But it is safe. Monolaurin is nontoxic to our bodies. According to every one of the studies, lauric acid is unsurpassed as a viral killer, and its monoglyceride form makes it even more effective than lauric acid alone.

Monolaurin, in particular, prevents and treats severe bacterial infections, especially those that are difficult to treat and antibiotic resistant. Monolaurin is used to inactivate measles, herpes simplex virus 1 and 2, and the herpes family members such as HIV, hepatitis C, vesicular, stomatitis virus (VSV), visna virus and cytomegalovirus.

Do you have a family member or friend who suffers from one of those and may have been told the condition is untreatable? Read him or her this chapter. And you saw the deadly HIV on the list. HIV isn't curable as yet, but it is treatable. Many of the pathogenic organisms inactivated by these antimicrobial lipids are also known to be responsible for opportunistic infections in HIV-positive individuals.

Take a look at this impressive list of infections worthy of attention by Monolaurin.

> **Monolaurin has been used to fight off:**
> - Newer, deadlier flu viruses (avian flu)
> - Strep throat
> - Staph infections
> - Respiratory Syctial Virus
> - Severe Acute Respiratory Syndrome
> - Ebola
> - Herpes Simplex Virus
> - Epstein-Barr Virus
> - Chronic Fatigue Syndrome
> - AIDS
> - Hepatitis C
> - Toxic Shock Syndrome
> - Fungi
> - Yeast infections
> - Protozoa parasites
> - Candida Albicans
> - Giardia
> - Chlamydia
> - Gonorrhea

A disclaimer is in order. To claim that Monolaurin can cure Ebola would be a foolish boast. So understand the difference between "treat" and "cure" and you will understand both the power and the limitation of this exceptionally versatile compound. Let's briefly explore a few of the uses Monolaurin has shown itself to exemplify...

Monolaurin helps immobilize Staph infection

Approximately 70% of bacteria that cause infections in hospitals are now resistant to those drugs most commonly used to treat infections. Difficult bacteria such as Staphylococcus aureus as well as other bacteria have been studied here in the United States in research groups such as Dr. H.G. Preuss's group at Georgetown University. Dr.Preuss found that Monolaurin inhibited pathogenic bacteria both in the petri dish (in vitro) and also in mice (in vivo).

Monolaurin rids your body of some pesky fungi, yeast, and protozoa

Monolaurin actually kills a great number of fungi, yeast, and protozoa parasites, such as ringworm, candida albicans, and the protozoan parasite Giardia lamblia, by the monoglycerides found in hydrolyzed human milk. In determining whether Monolaurin will be effective against a specific problem, someone afflicted with that problem should be sure the analysis is correct. Many ailments seem to be the same. (Note the discussion of Epstein-Barr a few paragraphs down, which points out how that virus often is confused with others producing parallel symptoms.)

Monolaurin pummels STDs.

Monolaurin has become extremely popular in treating rampant sexually transmitted diseases. Hydrogels containing Monocaprin and Monolaurin are powerful warriors when it comes to deactivating Chlamydia, gonorrhea, and HSV-2 and HIV-1. It's been shown to have anti-chlamydia and anti-gonorrhea effects in laboratory experiments with cell tissues. In a society in which sexually-transmitted diseases not only are rampant but a cause of social abhorrence, Monolaurin represents hope for the infected, who can have an opportunity to try a treatment that doesn't demand visits to a physician or being a social outcast. A peripheral benefit is that if a condition doesn't respond to Monolaurin, no harm ensues.

Monolaurin gives Epstein Barr the boot.

Similar protocols are used with Epstein Barr virus, which by the way, resembles the herpes virus. Epstein Barr is possibly responsible for Chronic Fatigue syndrome and quite possibly Multiple Sclerosis. Oh, you say, nobody you know has ever been infected with Epstein-Barr? Wrong. Epstein-Barr virus is one of the most common human viruses. It shows up in every country on every continent. In fact – and this is hard to believe if you haven't studied EBV – most people become infected with EBV sometime during their lives. And by most people I mean most people. In the United States, as many as 95 percent of adults between 35 and 40 years of age have been infected with EBV at some time during their lives. The reason we tend to think we've never had it is because EBV infections usually cause no symptoms or are indistinguishable from the other mild, brief illnesses of childhood. Infants become susceptible to EBV as soon as maternal antibody protection (present at birth) disappears. When infection with EBV occurs during adolescence or young adulthood, it causes infectious mononucleosis 35% to 50% of the time.

Are you feeling sick yet?

If you're sensing the early warning signs of the flu, sniffles, swollen glands or a scratchy throat, take the first line of defense: Monolaurin. Monolaurin is not something you need to take every day; but rather take it as a powerful anti-bacterial, or antiviral when you're feeling sick.

Antibiotic resistance has become a worldwide problem for treating infections caused by numerous organisms. Safe, effective antimicrobials that are not easily subject to resistance are desperately needed along with antiviral treatments. Monolaurin is beneficial as a nutritional supplement for microbial infections. The antimicrobial fatty acids and the derivatives are essentially nontoxic to humans.

We'll end this discussion of Monolaurin, one of the more controversial supplements discussed in this book, with a caution: Research isn't yet total. Research isn't yet complete. Research can be self-contradictory.

So it's possible you or a loved one can take Monolaurin caplets and not show the kind of improvement you hoped for. But even with that negative in place, a major positive is that no study has shown that Monolaurin can cause damage.

A great many expensive prescription remedies wish they could make that claim.

CHAPTER FIFTEEN

Probiotics

The truths and the myths of life-giving bacteria: Probiotics

Truth: "Probiotics will be to medicine in the 21st century what antibiotics and microbiology were in the 20th century." (Dr. Michael L. McCann)

What would you say if I told you that more bacteria live in your body at one time than there are people living on this earth? Here's what I'd say: "Yuck – where's the shower?"

Now, imagine this: Twenty times more bacteria live in our bodies (that number excludes viruses, yeasts, and parasites) than there are cells that make up who we are.

Not to worry. Less than one percent of these microorganisms are "germs" or uninvited guests.

Truth: Probiotics are life-giving bacteria

The bacteria bifidobacteria, along with lactobacilli, streptococci, clostridia, coliform and bacteriodes – belong to a group of bacteria called lactic acid bacteria – or Probiotics. These bacteria are considered "friendly" bacteria for a good reason: they're the gatekeepers who keep infections from penetrating our bodies. Cultivating a healthy balanced colony of these "friendly" bacteria is essential to living a healthy life.

What's considered healthy?

Proper balance of our digestive tract requires at least 85% "friendly" bacteria and not more than 15% harmful bacteria. Here's how it works: The food we eat is partially digested in the alimentary canal, mouth, stomach, and finally the intestines, where partially digested food is ultimately metabolized by billions of microorganisms (consisting of bacteria, yeasts, simple fungi, algae, protozoans) working together synergistically.

The down side: why bad bacteria are multiplying in our bodies

Don't worry, there's an upside too, and we'll get to that in a second. But here's some food for thought: During the technological revolution of the 20th century, we were blessed with wonder drugs: antibiotics. Now we know – and here's the downside – antibiotics are the number one cause of an imbalance in our bodies. A growing number of microorganisms have developed partial or total resistance to antibiotics.

The various foods we eat and use everyday are littered with second-hand antibiotics. What foods? How about meat, poultry and dairy products ... oral contraceptives ... steroids ... chlorinated water ... radiated items ... and refined sugars and other refined foods. Add to those elements such as poor digestion and/or poor elimination of waste. And be sure to add these: stress, and tension (the 21st century's favorite pastimes). All these factors contribute to our imbalance, with bad bacteria swamping good bacteria.

As we move deeper through the first decade of the 21st century we're bombarded with a hustle-and-bustle lifestyle that was unimaginable 30 years ago. Because of the way we live today, often without conscious choice, we need to pay special attention to ensure we have sufficient amounts of lactic acid bacteria vital to keeping our bodies healthy. We live our daily lives in a maelstrom of unhealthy conditions such as:

- Stress,
- Onset of disease,
- Ingestion of antibiotics and/or medications,
- Improper food and rest,
- Harmful environmental conditions.

These factors, not to mention improper diets, endanger the fine balance of our intestinal flora, preventing friendly bacteria from flourishing in our digestive tract.

The loss of Probiotics or lactic acid bacteria, and the subsequent appearance of detrimental microorganisms in the colon, both contribute to the production of endotoxins in the GI tract. That dangerous condition can lead to:

- Leaky bowel syndrome.
- Crohn's disease.
- Ulcerative colitis.
- Spastic colon.
- Irritable bowel syndrome.
- Autoimmune diseases.
- Overproduction of thyroid hormone.
- Candida albicans.
- Staphylococcus aureus.
- E. coli.
- Lupus erythematosus.
- Pacreatitis.

> *Health Notes: The people in the Balkans are known for their long, healthy lifespan due to eating large quantities of lactobacilli and other lactic organisms by way of fermented foods, which inhibit undesirable bacteria, and detoxify the system.*

- Psoriasis and other skin problems.
- Nervous system disorders.
- Rheumatoid arthritis.

My point isn't to put you in panic mode, but to give you an awareness of what can happen when the balance of our intestinal microflora is upset. Once the good/bad ratio of our intestinal bacteria gets thrown out of balance, you can bet that sooner or later, if left untreated, your intestinal tract is going to be infiltrated – make that invaded – by the "bad" bacteria, making it fertile ground for any one of these life-threatening maladies listed above.

The upside—keeping your intestines healthy with Probiotics

It's easy. It's natural. Probiotics counteract intestinal imbalances in our GI tract simply by proper diet and supplements. Probiotics (lactic acid bacteria) naturally benefit the body by maintaining a healthy balance of microflora in the intestinal tract and by acting directly on our intestinal cells. The benefits can vary depending on the dosage and type of Probiotic bacteria. Scientists are in total agreement that it's a necessity to be diligent in getting daily Probiotics to ensure the delicate balance of lactic acid bacteria your system.

A daily dose of high quality Probiotics containing both the twelve strains of viable lactic acid bacteria and high quality micronutrient byproducts is the most efficient way to restore and maintain bacterial balance in today's environment.

The discovery of Probiotic properties in fermented foods

You may think Probiotics is a relatively new idea. On the contrary, the theory that using "friendly" bacteria to improve our health dates back over 100 years when Russian physiologist and microbiologist Elie Metchnikoff was scorned by his colleagues for his offbeat theories.

In 1908, those same theories won Metchnikoff the Nobel Prize. Metchnikoff's work was first based on his observations of the Balkans in Eastern Europe – specifically, what the residents ate that enabled them to live long, healthy lives. He found the typical Balkan consumed large volumes of fresh yogurt … and lived a long, healthy life compared with people in other ethnic groups. Dr. Metchnikoff's theory of "good" bacteria was radical at the time but today, Probiotic supplements are sold in pharmacies, health food stores, and supermarkets around the world.

Another leader in Probiotics

Dr. Iichiroh Ohhira, Ph.D., renowned and award-winning microbiologist from Kayama University in Japan, also has dedicated his life to investigating and perfecting the science of Probiotic health by isolating the causes that constitute Probiotic balance and to ensure adequate colonies of "friendly" bacteria in the colon.

During his research, Dr. Ohhira (paralleling Metchnikoff, but working in Malaysia) found the evidence he was looking for in the difference between people with a history of longevity and good health versus those who did not. What he found from studying the diets of Malaysian people was how vitally important essential lactic acid bacteria is to the health of their bodies. His findings revealed that the Malaysian diet consisted of mainly fermented foods ripe with lactic acid bacteria. Both Metchnikoff and Ohhira concluded the same findings: Fermented foods filled with lactic acid bacteria help balance the body's intestinal tract.

The next logical step for Dr. Ohhira was to identify and isolate the beneficial ingredients of the fermented foods typically consumed in Asia. As Dr. Ohhira researched these foods over a period spanning two decades, he confirmed that although it's true that our bodies need 85% of the good bacteria for basic nourishment, of the several hundred kinds of lactic acid bacteria only about 20 strains are actually beneficial to our health.

The upshot: By balancing the beneficial and harmful bacteria that live naturally in our digestive tract, we maintain the number of beneficial bacteria and keep the population of potentially harmful bacteria in check. Ohhira's findings: Our bodies positively require different strains of lactic acid bacteria to break down our food, for nutrient absorption and even for producing certain vitamins to maintain the necessary eco-system our bodies need to survive.

Healthy Notes – be cautious of what you eat:

Although you can positively eat foods rich in "friendly bacteria" that naturally benefit your digestive tract, a nasty reality: Today, much of our food is riddled by second-hand exposure to antibiotics and pesticides, contraceptives, and steroids causing dysbiosis -- higher waste byproducts levels overburdening the body's waste removal mechanisms. which negates the growth and any existing "friendly" bacteria in our systems.

The myth: Ingesting large quantities of Probiotics will improve your digestive tract.

You might conclude, based on Dr. Ohhira's research, that if you provide your body with a large number of good bacteria it would lead to a dramatic improvement in the health of your digestive tract.

This conclusion would be wrong and would fool you into a false sense of health.

Why? Think about the cause and effect for a moment:

Cause: Too much stress, illness, ingestion of antibiotics and medicines, improper foods lack of rest, and harmful environmental conditions endangering the balance of intestinal flora.

Effects: An imbalance in the body's delicate eco-system. The inevitable result is inability to absorb vital nutrients in the GI tract. So logic prevails. If our GI tract can't absorb nutrients properly, we can't absorb the Probiotics our bodies so desperately need.

Dr. Ohhira found that the consumption and short-term presence of good bacteria alone doesn't lead to good health unless the digestive tract is free from the continual onslaught of harmful microorganisms including yeasts, viruses, and bad bacteria.

So then, in order for your body to benefit from Probiotics, the proper colonic pH balance needs to be reestablished in the body. Simply introducing friendly bacteria in large numbers will not resolve this imbalanced environment because the unfavorable colonic condition established in the system has become conducive only to proliferating more harmful microorganisms.

Bigger myth: All Probiotics are equal

As you'll see, not all Probiotics are created equal. Let's take a look at how they work:

History: Understanding the foundation of good health to be the balance of microflora in the colon, Dr. Ohhira concluded that a vital piece was missing: removing the harmful bacteria from the colon by creating an exclusive condition that not only puts friendly bacteria back into the system but creates a breeding ground for propagating more "friendly" bacteria, while eliminating and cleaning the intestinal tract from harmful bacteria for better absorption. Eradication of the harmful bacteria, of course, needs to be done in a natural manner.

The picture: "Friendly" bacterial colonization in the GI tract begins at birth. What Ohhira found was that a higher percent of children who were breast-fed enjoyed greater health and a stronger immune system compared against those infants who were not breast-fed. What he also observed was that while the breast-fed children acquired larger numbers of friendly strains of bifidobacteria, the children who weren't breast-fed produced a lesser amount or none at all. Scientists also agree that cesarean-section babies frequently have lesser amounts of friendly bacteria compared with normal birth babies. In some instances, the C-section babies lacked certain strains of good bacteria entirely. These findings led scientists to surmise that certain good bacteria are introduced to the infant as it passes through the mother's birth canal.

The breakdown: Acidic colon conditions of breast-fed babies remained within a constant range of pH 5.5 to 6.5. Studies demonstrated that the presence of sufficient levels of lactic acid in the colon of infants creates this healthy acidic condition. It's mainly the organic acids produced by the lactic acid bacteria present in the colon that prevent the survival of harmful bacteria in a baby's intestinal tract. This condition forms the first line of defense for the baby against disease.

The discovery: Dr. Ohhira (and other scientists as well) found that excessive use of antibiotics led to the creation of new strains of "smart" bacteria that have become resistant to antibiotics. To combat these new strains of bacteria Dr. Ohhira's team developed a special strain of friendly lactic acid bacteria that was isolated from the Malaysian culinary soy-based food – tempeh. Tempeh is a natural culturing and controlled fermentation process that binds soybeans into a cake form. Tempeh's fermentation process and its retention of the whole bean give it a higher content of protein, dietary fiber and vitamins. The bacterium, called the TH10 strain, was found to be highly effective when studied in vitro against the most potent antibiotic resistant MRSA smart bug, as well as E.coli (food poisoning), H. pylori (cause of peptic ulcers, morning sickness and migraines), Bacillus cereus (the cause of intestinal anthrax), and other harmful microorganisms.

Truth: TH10 is the definitive bacterial strain to ensure the elimination of harmful bacteria and toxins

Once the body ingests the TH10 bacteria, the bacteria begin to take hold in the GI tract, flourishing, and mingling with other strains of bacteria such as, lactobacillus and bifidobacteria strains. These good bacteria proliferate and aid in the digestion and, YES, the absorption of nutrients, while they form a barrier against the invasion of bad bacteria.

Dr. Ohhira's discovery led him to create an all natural, non-dairy, non-GMO vegetarian formula blend - a cornucopia of seaweeds, organic vegetables, herbs, fruits and leaves - plus the 12 strains of live lactic acid bacteria, including TH10, which provides the most prominent strain of bacteria possessing the highest proteolytic power in the world. (Proteolytics are enzymes that break the long chainlike molecules of proteins into shorter fragments (peptides) and eventually into their components, amino acids.) In fact, scientists have established that TH10 strain of lactic acid bacteria contained only in Dr. Ohhira's Probiotics is 6.25 times stronger than any other naturally occurring lactic acid bacteria. This blend is fermented and is inspected daily for pH and nutrient levels of the fermented product to guard against any contamination.

The better your GI tract balance, the better your health. If you consume any type of Western diet, chances are you suffer from microbial imbalances. I'm not about to ignore that. Are you?

I think we can all conclude the logical steps:
The first course of action is to ensure that we clear out the toxins that have formed in our digestive tracts so that we can start absorbing much needed nutrients again. The second course of action? It's obvious: to ensure these toxins are replaced with healthy, live-giving Probiotics.

CHAPTER SIXTEEN

Resveratrol

Resveratrol:
The power of the grape. The fruit of the gods.
And the promise of cellular health and longevity.

There's something to be said about a great French Bordeaux wine. It's more than its intoxicating aroma, and exquisite taste. One glass of wine contains an abundance of life-enriching enzymes and antioxidants – and a powerhouse nutrient called Resveratrol.

Today, Resveratrol is rocking the scientific world. Those who are touting its extraordinary benefits are among some very highly respected scientists from Harvard University and MIT. And, as we speak they're quite possibly doing battle over who's going to win the billion-dollar prize for creating the synthetic drug that mimics what Resveratrol does naturally for longevity.

This botanical, my friend, is making astounding headlines across the globe.

The history of the grape

The grape has certainly made its own decadent splash in history. Aptly named the "fruit of the gods" – the grape naturally contains this tiny fountain of youth called Resveratrol. Could it be the Greeks and the Romans were right in their folklore? That the grape is the "eternal" fruit of the gods and the reason why these legendary "gods" were purportedly immortal?

It's not the just the romance that makes this nutrient so alluring – it's the science that backs it up.

Where does Resveratrol come from?

Resveratrol can be found in grapes, raspberries, mulberries, blueberries, cranberries, peanuts and many species of pine. But the grape contains the highest concentrated levels of Resveratrol in its skin.

The grape is 50xs more potent in antioxidants than vitamin E and vitamin C, and loaded with Resveratrol that controls free radicals and prevents premature aging. (I know, you've heard that before – but there's one fact you haven't heard before – Resveratrol activates two newly discovered genes called SIRT genes that act as gatekeepers for cellular longevity and as inducers of the mechanism called "caloric restriction" initiated inside our cells.

In the news: Approximately 750 scientific reports on Resveratrol have been published stating the benefits of this miracle nutrient. To name a few:

- Revitalization of our cells
- Halts the signs of aging and promotes healthy aging
- Increases energy
- Reduces caloric intake and promotes healthy weight loss and diet
- Activates the newly discovered SIRT genes to increase the life our cells
- Protects our breast, prostrate, and endometrial tissues
- Helps our blood breathe and circulate smoothly
- Converts into an anti-cancer agent (selectively targeting and destroying cancer cells)
- Contains anti-viral properties
- Releases nitric oxide to prevent organ damage
- Reduces LDL cholesterol oxidation
- Inhibits inflammatory agents N Kappa B (which responds to stress)
- Inhibits Prostaglandin E-2 and Cox –2 enzymes (involved in cellular irritation)
- Protects us against sun damage to our skin
- Improves the health of our heart

My friend, here lies the key to cellular health and longevity. Resveratrol practically guarantees its promise of youthful vitality and long life.

Healthy aging – prolonged cellular life
Note: The important discovery linking Resveratrol's activation of two SIRT genes makes a heavy claim to prolong health and life by suppressing the common killers of age.

Let's take a look:
Headline news: "A supplemental component – Resveratrol is thought to lengthen the human life span by 70%, up to 50 years. A 125-year lifespan could become commonplace," says Dr. David Sinclair. Sinclair, (a pathology professor at Harvard Medical School).

Sinclair, along with Leonard Guarente of MIT, and scientists from Cornell Medical School and National Institutes of Health reported the discovery of SIRTS genes in our cells that act as gatekeepers for cellular longevity.

These newly discovered SIRT genes (sometimes called "survival genes") can purportedly be activated and placed in charge of cellular longevity.

The SIRTS genes increase the production of an enzyme that prolongs the time a living cell has to repair its DNA material. The enzyme is normally produced when the survival of living cells is threatened by starvation, germ exposure, or solar ultraviolet radiation.

Here's how it works: According to Dr. Sinclair's team, when the cells undergo caloric restriction signals sent through the membrane they activate a gene called NAMPT (nicotinamide phosphoribosyltransferase). As levels of NAMPT accelerate, a small molecule called NAD begins to amass in the mitochondria of the cell. This, in turn, causes the activity of enzymes created by the SIRTS genes to increase the enzymes that live in the mitochondria as well. The result: The mitochondria grow stronger, energy-output increases, and the cell's aging process slows down significantly.

"Mitochondria are the guardians of cell survival," explains Sinclair. "If we keep activating buckets of SIRTs into the mitochondria, then for a period of time the cell really needs nothing else.

Undoubtedly, Resveratrol can play an important role in cellular longevity and health for its known ability to activate the SIRT genes.

Resveratrol allows us to "cheat" on calories

SIRT genes are found to activate a mechanism in our cells called "caloric restriction". Resveratrol plays the role in activating these genes, which according to Dr. Sinclair negates the added effects of a high-fat diet in mice.

Here's what they found:

"Resveratrol shifts the physiology of middle-aged mice on a high-calorie diet towards that of mice on a standard diet and significantly increases their survival. Resveratrol produces changes associated with longer lifespan, including increased insulin sensitivity, reduced insulin-like growth factor-1 (IGF-I) levels, increased AMP-activated protein kinase (AMPK) and peroxisome proliferator-activated receptor activity, increased mitochondrial number, and improved motor function.

"Parametric analysis of gene set enrichment revealed that Resveratrol opposed the effects of the high-calorie diets in 144 out of 153 significantly altered pathways. These data show that improving general health in mammals using small molecules is an attainable goal, and point to new approaches for treating obesity-related disorders and diseases of ageing."

The researchers also found that low doses of Resveratrol activate SIRT genes which in turn mimic the effects of what is known as the "caloric restriction" and sends the message to our cells to start initializes a healthy low caloric intake. Diets with 20-30% fewer calories than a typical diet have been shown to extend the lifespan and blunt the effects of aging in numerous studies.

Caloric restriction reduces the energy load the body needs to break down a high fat and sugar diet. The more energy we conserve extends our lives. It does work. I've been on a 500-800 calorie diet for 5 weeks. I lost 20 pounds and I have plenty of energy. When I went back to 1500-2500 calories per day I could barely get up in the morning. This tells me my body is using all its energy to breakdown a heavier load of calories. I feel bloated and tired. One morning I couldn't even ride my bike to work which I do every day. I'm sticking with a lower calorie diet. My doctor couldn't even believe I kept all my muscle mass. I have 9% body fat.

The well-known fact that caloric restriction prolongs the life has been a scientific fact for over 70 years – however the prospect of nearly starving oneself certainly is not the number one choice for any sane person.

Now it seems people will no longer feel the need to starve themselves in order to prolong their lives. Why would they when they have something as natural as Resveratrol?

The culprits of premature aging

Let's break down the process of aging. At the core of the aging process are free radicals and oxidation and inflammation.

Free radicals are atoms or groups of atoms with an unpaired number of electrons that are formed when oxygen interacts with certain molecules. They attach to other molecules, causing our cells to become impaired.

Those molecules then become free radicals themselves, and the process keeps expanding wider, and wider.

Oxidation. The signs of normal aging – wrinkles, age spots, and loss of body function – can be partly attributed to the process of oxidation.

Inflammation: Resveratrol inhibits inflammatory agents like NF-Kappa B, a compound that "turns on" the inflammatory response. Halting these agents benefit our entire body – especially our heart.

Resveratrol's role in reducing the signs of aging

Antioxidants are molecules that can safely quench free radicals and halt the chain reaction of cellular damage. Resveratrol upgrades the body's antioxidant capacities. Studies show that it enhances the effectiveness of other antioxidants in the blood, such as vitamins C and E, or beta-carotene.

Most impressive, Resveratrol, like caloric restriction, may block the decline in heart function typically associated with aging. Professor Tomas Prolla, the senior researcher, stated: "Resveratrol at low doses can retard some aspects of the aging process, including heart aging, and it may do so by mimicking some of the effects of caloric restriction, which is known to retard aging in several tissues and extend life span." Additionally Prolla said, "Resveratrol is active in much lower doses than previously thought and mimics a significant fraction of the profile of caloric restriction at the gene expression level." Prolla also said, "I think there's a high likelihood that our findings are applicable to humans."

Suppressing cancer-causing agents

Researchers at the University of Rochester announced the results of a new study where Resveratrol kills pancreatic cancer cells while protecting healthy cells from radiation treatment; Resveratrol acts by disabling the cancer cell's mitochondria (i.e. its power source). According to the study's lead author, Dr. Paul Okunieff, "Resveratrol seems to have a therapeutic gain by making tumor cells more sensitive to radiation and making normal tissue less sensitive." According to Dr. Okunieff, "This research indicates that Resveratrol has a promising future as part of the treatment for cancer."

Dr. David Sinclair also shows that SIRT gene activation can suppress tumor formation and growth in the colon and intestine. A new study that confirms that over-expression of the SIRT1 enzyme can suppress tumor formation and growth in a preclinical mouse model of colon cancer. This is the first in-vivo data showing that SIRT1 can suppress tumor cell development. Resveratrol is a known activator of SIRT1. This is just another indication that Resveratrol may be used to prevent and fight cancer in the very near future.

Resveratrol may reverse potential problems of heart disease before the happen

Resveratrol works to combat potential problems of heart disease in three ways:

1. Resveratrol increases the health of the mitochondria.

Researchers at UCLA engineered mice to have defective mitochondria (the 'power plants' of the cell). In about half the normal time these mice developed heart disease. Scientists speculate that damaged and dying mitochondria are responsible for many diseases of aging - including heart disease, Alzheimer's disease, cancer, and diabetes. Studies have shown that Resveratrol can dramatically increase the number of mitochondria in cells.

2. Resveratrol inhibits inflammation.

Inflammation wreaks havoc on our hearts in quite a few ways. Studies show us that inflammation is one of the major causes of atherosclerosis because of its contributing factor in fatty deposits building in the lining of the arteries. Once these fatty deposits accumulate, arteries clog and can cause heart attacks and strokes. Resveratrol inhibits inflammatory agents like NF-Kappa B, a compound that "turns on" the inflammatory response. Halting these agents benefit our entire body – especially our heart.

3. Resveratrol keeps our blood breathing and circulating smoothly.

Our bodies have irregularly shaped cell fragments (blood platelets) that clot the blood when we need it to. These blood platelets can easily block a cerebral or coronary artery – another path that leads to heart attacks and strokes. Thankfully, Resveratrol inhibits blood platelets from aggregating.

5 to 10% of heart attack victims suffer a condition called atrial fibrillation, a fluttering of the top chambers of the heart. Atrial fibrillation also produces blood clots that can result in a stroke. In a recent study, Resveratrol was given to selected rodents before inducing a heart attack, the other rodents received nothing before the heart attacks were induced. The mortality rate of the rodents who received the Resveratrol was 10% and the fibrillation lasted an average of 112 seconds. Compare those stats to a 50% mortality rate and fibrillation lasting an average of 164 seconds for the rodents who received no Resveratrol.

I'd say, Resveratrol has the power to make everyone's heart happy.

Conclusion:

Incorporating Resveratrol into your daily routine is a wise strategy for healthy living in every aspect of your daily life. It's rare to find such natural nutrients with such phenomenal efficacy and potency. I know you'll benefit from its availability. I certainly do. What I recommend is Resveratrol 100 by Source Naturals. If you find something better you can let me know.

CHAPTER SEVENTEEN

Ribose

The Life Changing Power of D-Ribose

To stay healthy and active, our bodies need energy … lots of energy. The energy produced by each of the trillions of cells in our bodies keeps our hearts beating, our muscles contracting, our brains functioning to send signals to the far reaches of our bodies and to nerves carrying those signals to each of our organs to sustain life.

Our bodies produce and consume extraordinary amounts of energy. For example, an average heart contains less than one gram of energy. But every day our hearts consume almost 6,000-grams of energy, pumping blood and delivering life-giving oxygen to tissues throughout our bodies. Think about the magnitude of this feat! Six-thousand grams is more than 10 times the average weight of a heart and almost 10,000 times the amount of energy that is normally found in the heart at any one time.

Ask yourself, "Where does this energy come from?" and "How can the heart produce such an extraordinary volume of energy?" In large part, the answers to these questions all are found in D-Ribose.

ATP – the currency of life

Virtually all the energy used by our bodies comes from a small molecule with a large name, Adenosine triphosphate, or simply ATP. In each cell, ATP is made, consumed, and re-processed in a cycle that keeps a continual supply of energy flowing. Our bodies have developed very elaborate metabolic processes to make sure we don't run out. These processes efficiently recycle energy as it is used, making fresh energy constantly available to sustain life. ATP has three basic parts. The first is D-Ribose, commonly simply called Ribose. Ribose provides the structural foundation upon which ATP is built and starts the process of ATP synthesis in the body. Without Ribose ATP could not be formed and our cells would be energy starved.

As long as we stay reasonably physically fit, and our cells get the oxygen they need to fuel metabolism, this cycle of energy utilization and supply can keep turning unimpeded. The problem comes when our cells are unable to get enough oxygen to keep the process flowing. Case in point: heart conditions affect how well the heart functions, and, therefore how efficiently it can deliver blood and oxygen to our tissues.

Many non-disease conditions also affect blood flow or oxygen delivery. As we age, for example, tissues lose their ability to use oxygen efficiently. Older tissue has a harder time keeping up the continual demand for energy. Even strenuous exercise can impact the relationship between energy supply and demand. When cells and tissues are unable to get the oxygen they need to maintain the balance of energy supply and demand, the results are fatigue, muscle pain, stiffness and soreness, reduced ability to exercise, and lower quality of life.

Putting gas in your tank

Supplying energy to your cells parallels keeping gasoline in your car. When your car is sitting in the garage with a full tank of gas it is fully fueled and ready for a long drive. When you start the car and head it down the road, though, you begin to consume the gas in the tank and the supply of energy gets progressively lower until you have to fill the tank with gas or you'll run out fuel and the engine will stop, leaving you stranded by the side of the road. The same thing is true in your body. When you have enough food and oxygen to supply energy your engine will keep running and you never will run out of gas. But if you can't get enough oxygen to keep the cell's energy tank fully fueled you progressively lose energy until you run out of gas. Then, you have to refill your tank before you can start down the road of life once more.

If you're healthy, you can refill your tank simply by resting long enough for new energy fuel to fill your cells. In a normal, healthy person who has strenuously exercised over a few days in a row, it takes more than three days of rest for cells to fully recharge. (This is typical of young athletes who might exercise every day. Frequently, these athletes don't let their bodies rest long enough to restore lost energy and, in a short time, they become fatigued, sore, stiff, weak, and out of sorts. They simply try to do too much work with too little fuel … and run out of gas.)

As we age, or if we suffer with heart or muscle disease, in contrast to the athlete performing strenuous exercise, the normal course of daily activities might be enough to fully consume the energy in our cells and tissues. As a result of running out of fuel we might become persistently or chronically fatigued. We could have leg soreness and muscle stiffness. We frequently can't face the prospect of climbing stairs or even walking out to the mailbox. We may be too tired to go shopping or to play with the grandchildren. And our quality of life suffers as a result. To make matters worse, our bodies might never deliver enough oxygen to let our cells fully recover once the energy in our cells and tissues is fully consumed.

Whether it is an athlete that wants to recover more quickly so they can get back on the field, an aging grandparent who longs for the energy to take the grandchildren to the park, an active professional with too much work, too much stress, and too little sleep, or a heart patient who can't face the prospect of climbing the stairs to bed, the issue is replacing fuel in the tank. Like the fuel pump at the gas station, Ribose is the metabolic fuel the body uses to recharge the energy batteries and put gas back in the tank.

The recovery power of Ribose

Replacing the energy that drains from our cellular gas tanks begins with Ribose. Our cells use this simple carbohydrate to initiate ATP synthesis, allowing our bodies to rebuild lost energy and recharge the cellular batteries. Every cell in our bodies makes Ribose every day. The problem is that our cells lack the metabolic machinery they need to make very much Ribose, or to make it quickly when our bodies need it. Our cells make Ribose from a very abundant and highly important carbohydrate called glucose, also known as dextrose. In the body, glucose is used as the primary metabolic fuel for many cellular reactions, and because of its importance it is rationed. This rationing prevents very much glucose from moving down the metabolic pathway to make Ribose. So when our bodies are stressed by strenuous exercise, metabolic dysfunction, or disease our cells can't recover until enough Ribose is made to stimulate ATP synthesis and refill our energy fuel tank. If our cells are aging or not functioning normally, we aren't able to supply enough oxygen to our tissues, or we don't allow ourselves sufficient rest, there might never be enough time to make an adequate amount of Ribose for our energy batteries to recharge.

Because the heart beats continually, it can't rest while its energy tank is refilled. Instead, the heart slows down certain energy consuming functions, conserving the energy left in its tank for contraction. The energy-starved heart tries its best to push blood and oxygen to the body, but because it does not have enough energy its efforts are inefficient and inadequate. As time goes on, this inefficient blood flow to the rest of the body begins to take a toll. As heart disease progresses, for example, patients may complain of overwhelming fatigue, shortness of breath, sore legs, or an inability to perform even simple exercise, such as walking up stairs or around the block.

The same is true of people with fibromyalgia or other neuromuscular disease affecting muscle metabolism. As in ischemic heart disease, this metabolic insufficiency drains the energy fuel tank leaving the muscle energy starved. This chronic and persistent energy drain forces a series of cellular reactions ending in muscle pain, soreness, stiffness, and fatigue. Patients with fibromyalgia, for example, often are too fatigued to maintain normal interaction with their friends or family, and may have too much pain to stay active or even keep their jobs. In many cases, these patients must be treated with anti-depressants because of the psychological stress inflicted by their illness, and in virtually every case doctors treat patients with pain pills that don't treat the underlying cause of the disease.

Supplying these affected tissues with Ribose stimulates the process of energy recovery and helps hearts and muscles refill their energy tanks. Supplemental Ribose allows cells to bypass the slow process of natural Ribose synthesis and accelerates ATP recovery. It doesn't matter whether we are talking about hearts or muscles, if we are healthy or sick, or if we are old or young. Cells need energy, and Ribose is fundamentally required to restore this lost energy and put the energy demand and supply ratio back in balance.

Two recent clinical studies have shown that Ribose supplementation can help patients overcome their shortness of breath and tolerate more exercise. Patients are able to breathe more efficiently and can utilize oxygen more effectively. The net result is that patients can do more exercise before running out of breath, and this directly impacts quality of life.

How do I know I need Ribose?

At some point in his or her life, everyone needs Ribose. We all face situations where Ribose supplementation could help us overcome the pain and stiffness of muscle overexertion, the fatigue of chronic disease, the weakness after strenuous exercise, or the inability to do the things we want to do. We all want to be as active and healthy as we can, and we need a full supply of energy in all our cells and tissues to reach that goal.

Although Ribose is made naturally in all our cells and tissues, it is a slow process. And this delay limits the speed with which our bodies can restore lost energy. Ribose is the limiting factor in ATP synthesis, and our bodies have an absolute and fundamental need for ATP to fuel the multitude of biochemical reactions that keep us alive and vital.

It's easy to determine who should take Ribose, and when. Anyone with a highly active lifestyle, for example, can certainly benefit from Ribose. High-intensity athletics three or more times per week puts a severe strain on hearts and muscles. Repeated bouts of strenuous exercise drains energy from hearts and muscles, leaving them weakened for the next exercise bout. When athletes take Ribose before, during, and after exercise, they can better maintain the energy in their muscles and quickly restore any energy that may have been lost.

Someone who is normally sedentary might face several days of muscle soreness, stiffness, and weakness following a day of hard work in the garden or a weekend softball game. Others who might be a little older or perhaps have problems with their circulation may complain of sore legs after only a short walk or a day of shopping. No matter where you fall along this spectrum, what is happening in your muscle is the same: Your muscle is consuming available energy, and that energy drain translates to weak, spongy, and sore muscles. This muscle soreness does not go away until the muscle has recovered its energy balance. Ribose supplementation helps maintain the muscle's energy balance and can be the answer to relieving this post-exertional muscle soreness and stiffness.

Age is another factor to consider when deciding if Ribose supplementation is right for you. Aging muscle generally has fewer of the energy recycling powerhouses, called mitochondria, than younger muscle. Continual loss of mitochondria as we age makes it more likely our muscles will run out of energy with less exertion. This is a primary reason that, when we become older we become stiff and sore after only mild exercise, and explains why we run out of gas so quickly. Also, as we age our hearts begin to show more and more signs of dysfunction. A recent research report from the Mayo Clinic, for example, showed that almost 25% of the population, both male and female, showed signs of heart failure, and the percentage increased as people grew older. While this effect was more pronounced in people with high blood pressure or in those with heart valve problems, it was found across the aging population. Taking Ribose regularly may help relieve the chronic muscle soreness and stiffness that comes from even mild exercise and, as has been shown in many clinical studies, could help maintain healthy energy levels in the heart.

We also need to include patients with heart disease when considering who should take Ribose. Research has proven, without doubt, that heart disease drains the heart of much needed energy. It is important that people with heart disease take Ribose regularly to offset the effects of energy drain in their hearts.

Patients with diseases that impact muscle metabolism should also seriously consider Ribose supplementation. Diseases such as fibromyalgia, chronic fatigue syndrome, myoadenylate deaminase disease, and McArdle's disease, for example, drain energy from muscles, and this energy drains shows itself in the form of fatigue, muscle pain, soreness, and stiffness. Ribose helps offset the all these symptoms.

Most of us don't know we have a problem with the energy in our hearts and muscles until we get sore legs, worn out, or chronically fatigued. But even after these symptoms hit us, it isn't too late. Ribose supplementation can quickly help replace energy in stressed hearts and muscles, and help maintain the normal energy balance in our tissue.

How much Ribose should I take?

Virtually any amount of Ribose you can give to stressed hearts and muscles will help. The amount of Ribose you should take is really dependent on what you want it to do. For example, if you simply want to give your heart and muscles a little boost, you can get by with less. If you want to increase your athletic performance, reduce soreness and stiffness following exercise, or give your muscles a recovery boost after some strenuous work or exercise, you might need a little more. And if you have heart disease, peripheral vascular disease, or other chronic conditions that impact energy metabolism in your heart or muscles, more aggressive supplementation may be required. Suggestions on dosage:

- **2 to 5 grams** (about one-half to one slightly rounded teaspoonful of powder) daily to help hearts and muscles maintain a healthy energy pool.

- **5 to 7 grams** (about one level to slightly rounded tablespoonful of powder) every day as a preventative in cardiovascular disease, for athletes who want to recover faster from high-intensity exercise, and for healthy people doing strenuous work or activities that are outside their normal level of daily exercise.

- **7 to 10 grams** daily for most patients with heart disease or peripheral vascular disease, for patients recovery from heart surgery or heart attack, and for athletes who work out frequently in high-intensity activities.

- **10 to 15 grams** daily for patients with more advanced heart disease, patients awaiting heart transplant, and patients with fibromyalgia or neuromuscular disease.

Daily doses should not be taken at once. Actually, smaller more frequent doses are better than larger less frequent doses. Although there are no safety concerns with taking Ribose (it is, after all, a simple carbohydrate), don't take more than 20-grams per day. (Once they give their hearts and muscles a chance to regain their energy balance, most people stabilize at about 10-grams per day.)

It generally takes no more than a few days to feel the effect of Ribose supplementation. If you don't begin to feel a positive effect after two or three days, try increasing the dose. The sickest patients usually feel the greatest benefit, but almost everyone taking Ribose regularly reports a significant benefit. Remember that your energy drain is chronic and Ribose can't be stored in your cells and tissues. Therefore, if you stop taking Ribose you will lose all the benefit you've gained and your heart or muscles will again become energy starved. So take Ribose every day and keep on taking it.

Ribose is found in many product forms, such as powders, beverages, nutrition bars, and tablets. As a practical matter, therapeutic levels are found only in powders. The most reputable supplier is Bioenergy Life Science (Minneapolis, MN), the leading contender in the world of Ribose research. All the safety data supplied to regulatory agencies has come from this company. These safety assessments have shown that Ribose is 100% safe if taken as directed and manufactured according to the strict specifications of Bioenergy Life Science.

There are very few reports of side effects while taking Ribose. Some people have reported being light-headed if they take doses greater than 10-grams on an empty stomach. That is why label instructions suggest that Ribose be taken with juice or another beverage containing additional carbohydrate. Sprinkling Ribose on fruit or cereal is also a good way to take it; or, if taken with a meal, it can be mixed with water, tea, or coffee. A mild side effect reported by people taking large doses is loose stools or mild diarrhea. This is common with any carbohydrate that absorbs water. Neither side effect is significant, and neither is found when Ribose is taken as directed. Ribose is also safe to take with your usual medicine and with other nutritional therapies. No drug or nutritional interactions with Ribose supplementation have been reported. Tens of thousands of people now take Ribose every day. Ribose stands alone as a nutrient that can increase the energy level in hearts and muscles and restore energy depleted by over-exertion or disease. No other compound, whether drug or other nutrient, can do what Ribose does in the body. Only Ribose can accelerate the complex metabolism that restores energy in our bodies, making it one of the most profound nutrients ever to be introduced.

CHAPTER EIGHTEEN

Vinpocetine

Vinpocetine:
The new brain rejuvenator

If you want to keep your mind sharp and your brain young -- toss out the Ginkgo Biloba -- and make room for Vinpocetine. Simply put, Vinpocetine is one of the most potent brain foods ever discovered. It actually helps keep the mind from faltering.

Ask yourself this: wouldn't you like to...
1. Improve your brainpower?
2. Improve your mental clarity and alertness?
3. Improve your concentration skills?
4. Increase your learning speed and ability to process information faster?
5. Improve your neuro-muscular coordination and your reaction time?
6. Improve your vision due to poor blood circulation to the eyes?
7. Improve your ability to remember and retrieve old memories?

Unless you're willing to settle for being less than you can be, this chapter will be of great importance in answering, "Yes!" To every one of those questions.

The Super Herb: Vinpocetine
The leaves of the periwinkle plant (vinca minor) give us the gift of Vinpocetine.

Its powerful curative abilities make it a powerhouse for combating the effects of cerebrovascular disorders (how blood circulates through the brain), memory loss in cases of Alzheimer's disease, and even mild dementia related to the normal aging process. Not only is it used for treating medical maladies, but it's good for everyone who wants the edge to be on top of their game by improving concentration, learning speed, and alertness.

What does that mean for you?
The research and its tested claims on Vinpocetine are nothing short of incredible. Vinpocetine not only improves memory and reduces memory loss by increasing your power to concentrate and retain information, but also acts as a healing agent for various disorders related to the functioning of our brains, such as, cerebral hemorrhage, strokes, senile dementia, transient ischemic attacks, and chronic cerebral circulatory insufficiencies. (Those terms may seem formidable. That's because the damage they can do to your brain really *is* formidable.)

How does Vinpocetine work?

Anyone over the age of 40 runs the risk of arteriosclerosis (hardening of the arteries). When fatty calcium deposits accumulate and harden in our arterial walls, the arteries narrow and restrict the blood flow. This disease develops gradually over a lifetime. But by the time serious symptoms develop to a point where they are recognized, the clogged blood vessels are usually well advanced. Vinpocetine minimizes structural and functional damage to the brain neurons, damage that may accompany developing cerebral arteriosclerosis.

Vinpocetine also benefits those who suffer from, or are at risk, of various brain functioning disorders such as cerebral hemorrhage, stroke, dementia, transient ischemic attacks (not getting enough blood flow to the brain), and chronic cerebral circulatory insufficiency. Vinpocetine is the safe brain metabolism enhancer a cognition-activating "smart drug." (Now, don't let that appellation fool you.) Vinpocetine isn't a drug, and that means it won't stir up the nasty side effects so many prescription drugs cause.

The importance of fueling your brain

Fueling oxygen to the brain, along with its primary fuel – glucose – is vitally important for producing 15-20% ATP, (the main energy source that the brain needs to run properly).

Imagine this: Your brain typically contains 10-100 billion neurons (electrically active nerve cells), and 10 times as many glial cells, (structural and nutritional support cells that surround the neurons). Your brain normally receives 15-20% of your body's total blood supply and will use 15-20% of your body's total inhaled oxygen.

Which means what? It means that unlike most other cells, which burn either fat or sugar for their energy, these neurons can only burn glucose under normal, non-starvation conditions. When neurons are oxygen starved, a different form of sugar burning occurs – anaerobic glycolysis – (without oxygen). When glucose brain fuel is burned without adequate oxygen only 5% of ATP energy is produced, as compared to when glucose is burned with a good quantity of oxygen.

> **Food for thought:**
> A study showed that Vinpocetine increased the ATP levels in red blood cells, which, in turn, resulted in better stimulation, release, and absorption of oxygen by hemoglobin in vascular dementia patients.

Okay, so what happens when these irreplaceable, life-essential neurons aren't receiving their proper blood supply and oxygen? They starve. They start to die. Why? These neurons consume 50% of the body's total blood sugar and are dependent upon a continuous and uninterrupted blood supply to maintain normal energy metabolism and avoid injury or death.

Vinpocetine counteracts the effects that cause the death of precious brain cells

When Vinpocetine was developed in the late 1960s, they found that the Vinpocetine compound improves blood flow to the brain, boosts brain cell ATP production (which is the main energy source for cellular function), and increases the amount of glucose and oxygen ushered into the neurons. For almost 30 years Vinpocetine has been used clinically to treat cerebrovasular (the blood circulation to the brain) disorders and symptoms related to aging due to cognitive deficiencies caused by hypoxia (insufficient oxygen to the brain), and ischemia (insufficient blood flow), assisting in bringing oxygen and glucose to the brain.

Science or science fiction?

In our country, why do you suppose the medical science field continually ignore the effects of life-enhancing nutrients? One can only speculate.

> *Food for thought…*
> *Clinical research in humans and animals now shows us that Vinpocetine restores impaired brain carbohydrate and energy metabolism.*

Science has been telling us that the brain peaks its total number of neurons at birth to 2 years of age. After that, they simply don't reproduce, so maintaining neuron health is extremely important to us. Some sources claim neurons not only stop reproducing themselves but also, as we age, slowly begin to die out.

Don't believe it… Today, ongoing research supports Vinpocetine as the hyper-booster for cerebral blood flow and neuron protection. These studies show that Vinpocetine can actually recover 25% of its neurons in areas where the brain has suffered from cellular death. Hard to believe? Studies confirm it.

Proof positive:
B. Vamosi and other experiments

I'm going to point out just a few of the hundreds of reports and studies proving Vinpocetine may safely and effectively help metabolize neuronal energy, even under hypoxic (insufficient oxygen flow) and ischemic (poor blood flow) conditions.

Until Vinpocetine arrived on the scene, Xanthinol Nicotinate was the champion in maintaining blood flow to the brain. Xanthinol Nicotinate is a highly potent form of Niacin, and everyone who ever has taken Niacin knows it can cause - flushing and itching. So where Xanthinol Nicotinate traditionally had been the popular choice for improving the reaction speed of the elderly, Vinpocetine, is the new champion.

In 1976, when B. Vamosi and his colleagues reported outstanding results in favor of Vinpocetine, when comparing it with Xanthinol Nicotinate in treating 143 patients with various cerebrovascular diseases. They found Vinpocetine to be the more superior of the two.

Here's how they did it:
They took a number of blood and cerebrospinal fluid variables such as glucose, lactate, pyruvate, oxygen, pH, and electrolyte levels before and after treating these variables with Vinpocetine and Xanthinol Nicotinate.

This is what they reported:
"Though not all the changes are significant statistically, yet when they're connected with each other, they prove that Vinpocetine enhances both the glycolytic and oxidative reactions of glucose breakdown in the brain. *"The changes in the concentration of potassium and magnesium may be considered a sign of recovery of the energy metabolism of the nerve cells."*

The neuro-regenerator
When researchers (Miyamoto, M, et al) studied the antioxidant effects on glutamate-damaged tissue, they discovered that Vinpocetine rids the brain of neuronal related injuries. This confirmed that Vinpocetine is in fact a strong neuro-protective agent proving to be 100 times more effective than Dilantin against drug-induced cell loss. Yes, you're reading right – *100 times* more effective.

Karpati and Szporny
Ready for some tech-talk? OK … when researchers Karpati and Szporny studied the repeated effects of low levels of oxygen to the brain (hypoxia), they reported that short-lived and partial interference with normal brain circulation caused a substantial increase of neuro-chemical disturbances (a chemical that naturally occurs in the nervous system), plus it showed that the oxygen process lacked formation mainly due to the oxygen shortage to the brain. These findings showed that mitochondrial metabolism (the principal energy source of the cell that converts nutrients into energy) failed to metabolize.

The good news: When Karpati and Szporny introduced Vinpocetine to the mix, it showed that it safely and effectively restored the mitochondrial energy metabolism, even under hypoxic or ischemic (poor blood flow) conditions.

Solti and the cerebral circulation

F. Solti and his colleagues created a study of ten men (average age 49), suffering from cerebrovascular disorders. At the conclusion of the study they agreed: "Vinpocetine belongs to a small select group of nutrients that exert a powerful effect on the cerebral circulation."

Solti concludes that Vinpocetine effects cerebral circulation in two ways:

1. Vinpocetine reduces the chance of poor blood flow that puts you at a high risk for strokes.

2. Vinpocetine does not affect blood pressure so it's very safe to use if you're taking medications for high blood pressure. Since this nutrient reduces the effort the it takes for the heart to output - rather than increasing its effort, Vinpocetine helps to improve blood flow Without causing undue stress on the heart and circulatory system.

> **Benefits at a glance:**
>
> • Restores long term mories.
>
> • Enhances cognitive function.
>
> • Increases mental alertness.
>
> • Combats structural and functional damage to the brain.
>
> • Enhances brain metabolism.

The difference between natural Vinpocetine and other cerebral vasodilators

Solti and other researchers concluded:
Vinpocetine is a unique selective cerebral vasodilator. It's selective because it does not open up the blood vessels in brain regions that don't suffer from reduced circulation.

Additional validating research came from:

Hadjieve and Yancheva
Vinpocetine hones and selects ONLY areas where blood supply is strangled in the brain.

Hadjieve and Yancheva, working with 50 patients suffering from impaired cerebral circulation, found their clinical results outstandingly in favor of

Vinpocetine. Their conclusions:

- Vinpocetine allows more blood supply only to parts of the brain that are injured. That making it 100 times more effective than other vasodilators that can't distinguish an injured part of the brain from a non-injured area.

- Non-selective vasodilators open up blood vessels in brain regions that don't suffer from reduced circulation more than opening blood vessels in regions suffering from damaged circulation. This occurrence can only be labeled as dangerous. Dangerous because this "steal effect" can cause a net shift of cerebral blood flow away from the injured area, causing further damage to the blood starved part of the brain. So, it's only natural to say that Vinpocetine is an excellent supplement choice compared to other non-selective vasodilators.

Can you prevent your brain from age-degeneration?

More tech-talk, but it's important. Vinpocetine reduces the effects of aging on the brain because of the starring role it plays with the noradrenaline nerve cluster in the Reticular Activating System called the "locus ceoruleus".

The locus coeruleus is a nucleus located in the brain stem. These valuable neurons innervate the cerebral cortex as well as the spinal cord, the brain stem, the cerebellum, hypothalamus, the thalamic relay nuclei, the amygdale, and the basal telencephalon.

Think of the locus ceoruleus neurons as the "mediators"of the sympathetic effects of stress. When they're activated by stressors, they'll secrete noradrenaline or norepinephrine through the nerve fibers to the cerebral cortex and increase cognitive function and motivation.

You can guess what happens as we age… the locus ceoruleus neurons decline increasingly with age. The outcome: concentration, alertness, and the ability to process information are trapped in the mind. The degeneration advances slightly faster in men than in women.

The Reticular Activating System gained the attention of neuroscientists interested in pathological conditions affecting behavior, such as Alzheimer's Disease.

An imbalance of norepinephrine in the cells of the Reticular Activating System is also thought to cause ADD and ADHD.

Olpe and his colleagues show us that Vincamine (as stated, also part of the periwinkle herb) and Vinpocetine are among the most effective means to re-activate the neurons in the locus coeruleus, making Vinpocetine a true cognition enhancing stimulator and something to celebrate.

EEG findings on the effects of aging

Saletu and Grunberger, known for their pioneering studies on the effects of drugs on EEG recordings, report, "Human brain function as measured by electroencephalogram (EEG) shows significant alterations in normal and pathological aging characterized by an increase of delta (slow wave) and theta activity and a decrease of alpha and beta activity (fast wave), as well as by slowing of the dominant EEG frequency."

These changes are indicative of deficits in the "vigilance regulatory systems," (which include the locus ceoruleus neurons). By the term vigilance we mean the dynamic state of total neural activity. Elderly subjects with bad memory exhibit slower EEG activity and less alpha and alpha-adjacent beta activity than those with good memory. Antihypoxidotic/nootropic drugs such as Vinpocetine induce, interestingly, oppositional changes to the age related slowing of EEG waves in human brain function, thereby improving vigilance. (Man's ability to adapt).

> *Food for thought:*
> *Micro-vessels that feed neurons in the brain and retina of the eye are smaller in diameter than a single red blood cell. These vessels can become easily clogged and impair local microcirculation. Vinpocetine prevents the blood from clotting up in the tiny blood vessels in the eyes.*

Is Vinpocetine safe to use?

No adverse effects have been found using Vinpocetine. Both human and animal studies show that the safety factor is remarkable.

However, I would advise speaking to your doctor before taking Vinpocetine. If you are, trying to get pregnant, or think you may be pregnant, you should probably not take Vinpocetine without strict monitoring.

What is the correct dosage for taking vinpocetine?

The typical dosage is 15-30mg a day.

Everybody ages… but wouldn't you rather do it knowing you'll have a better quality of life?

If you're like most people, you want to keep your mind sharp and your brain young and you want to keep the super power your brain was meant to have. You have the power to help prevent the degeneration and inherent diseases that go along with an aging brain.

I'm going to suggest that Vinpocetine is the "smarter," and safer food for your thoughts and comprehension. I can't imagine anyone saying no to that.

CHAPTER NINETEEN

Wheat Grass

The Power of Wheatgrass:
A bounty of nutrients for vibrant health

We've all heard a version of this tune before: "If you want dessert – eat your vegetables." Did we listen? I know I didn't. And according to this statistic, not many of us did: Research tells us that as Americans, our diets mainly consist of an intake of 2,000 to 3,000 calories a day made up from dairy products, refined flours, cereals and sugars, refined vegetable oils, meat and alcohol. To add insult to bodily injury - only 3 to 5% of the calories come from eating fruits and vegetables.

As a result of the average diet, most of us ultimately suffer from one of more of these ailments in our lifetime:

Arthritis	High blood pressure
Respiratory problems	Anemia
Low energy	Skin rashes
Prostate problems	Kidney stones
Sleeping disorders	Body odor
Panic Attacks	Poor vision
Sinusitis	Headaches/Migraines
Diabetes	Poor metabolism
Ulcers	Immune disorders
Muscle pain	Hair loss
Parasites	High cholesterol
Heart disease	Epileptic seizure
Gastrointestinal problems	Dental problems
Menstrual, & Menopausal symptoms	Cancers/Tumors

Merely treating these symptoms is a cover-up. Prevention is the key. Here's how:

Your body requires one and a half to two pounds of vegetables – Every Day!

That's 3-5 servings a day. Some of the most important types of vegetables are the dark leafy green vegetables. And yet, I would wager that more than 50% of the people in America don't plan their meals around their vegetables.

What are the best sources of dark leafy vegetables?

Look for a deep green color and the thickness of the leaves. Kale and Wheatgrass are the richest in nutrients compared to other leafy green vegetables. Kale is one of the hardiest leafy green vegetables. Its green color is one of the deepest and its leaves are not thin but thick and strong. Spinach is dark green but has a less hardy constitution. Its leaves are thin and wilt easily. Wheatgrass is considered a dark green leafy vegetable with a long history of being one of the strongest natural sources of nutrients.

The abundant properties of Wheatgrass
Wheatgrass is one of the simplest foods, and one of the most abundantly rich in health-enriching nutrients.

But there's a catch: Wheatgrass contains a high amount of cellulose (tough fiber) that affects the availability of its nutrients. You see, unlike other animals, we have a hard time digesting cellulose for optimum nutrient delivery.

Because of this, the best way to take full advantage of nutrient-rich Wheatgrass is by its juice.

Here's why: Our stomachs weren't made to break down cellulose fiber efficiently.
The cellulose contained in the whole-ground grass can actually halt the delivery of some of its nutrients. Our bodies can assimilate the juice immediately because it dissolves in our mouths rather than going through the long digestive process and losing the nutrients. Those of us with slow or problematic digestion benefit from the easy assimilation factor of the juice, and get the benefits of its pure unadulterated nutrients.

Wheatgrass juice delivers a bounty of vitamins
1. Vitamin K. Those who suffer from vitamin K deficiencies most often have chronic diarrhea, liver diseases, pancreas disease or cystic fibrosis. Lack of this vitamin results in prolonged bruising and prolonged bleeding from small injuries. Studies are finding that Vitamin K deficiency can be a contributing factor in developing Alzheimer's disease. Vitamin K may also help play a role preventing osteoporosis, atherosclerosis, arthritis, and diabetes by its ability to aid bone strengthening, and keeping calcium from the linings of arteries.

We often lose Vitamin K by the chronic use of mineral oil products internally, as well as aspirin and antibiotics. Low fat diets can also deplete this vitamin, as well as a digestive tract with a high amount of bad bacteria. Unlike synthetic Vitamin K, which in excessive amounts has been proven to be toxic, the natural Vitamin K, found in Wheatgrass juice and dark green leafy vegetables, is non-toxic in any amount.

2. Vitamin A: Wheatgrass juice is high in beta-carotene, which converts to Vitamin A. It's not known to be toxic in any amount, although the skin can become an orange color if you consume vast amounts.

3. Vitamin C: Wheatgrass juice is great a source of Vitamin C. Lack of Vitamin C shows up as a weak structure in blood cells, skin, gums, bones and connective tissue because the protein collagen can't form when there's a deficiency of Vitamin C.

4. Folic Acid: Women using birth control pills or alcoholics usually suffer from folic acid deficiency. It shows up as anemia, irritability, gas, bloating, and sores in the corners of the mouth. Wheatgrass juice is a good source for the daily requirements of Folic Acid.

5. B12: B-12 found in Wheatgrass is required for folic acid conversion and for the formation of nucleic acids – a group of complex acids occurring in all living cells, RNA and DNA, new tissues and red blood cells. In order to absorb B12 the body also needs B-6 and calcium, which are also found in Wheatgrass juice.

6. Protein: It's commonly known that plant protein is much easier than most animal protein to digest. Wheatgrass juice contains all essential and non-essential amino acids.

Green leaf protein in most Wheatgrass and wheatgrass juice powder is anywhere from 9% - 25%. I recommend Sweet Wheat® Organic Wheatgrass Juice Powder because it contains 30% and can be as high as 40% per serving size of protein.

Here's a comparison of common foods and their percentage of protein per serving in comparison:
>   4 oz. (113 grams) yogurt = 10% protein
>   1 egg   (50 grams) = 10% protein
>   1 oz. (28 grams) fresh mozzarella = 18% protein
>   4 oz. (112 grams) organic ground beef = 19% protein
>   1 cup (8 oz.) organic milk = 8 grams protein
>   1-1/2 grams Sweet Wheat = 30-40% per serving of protein

Dr. James Balch, M.D., a physician and surgeon for over thirty-five years and leading authority on integrative medicine and nutritional healing, states: "Wheatgrass juice is the 'King of Juices' – one ounce is equal to a pound and a half of fresh vegetables. It's rich in vitamins A, C, and E, as well as calcium, phosphorus, iron, potassium, cobalt and zinc. And best of all it's rich in chlorophyll, the substance that 'purifies the blood, suppresses bacterial growth and counteracts toxins."

The history of Wheatgrass
Wheatgrass comes from the wheat plant. Wheat of course, has been used as a staple in our diets for centuries. Wheat is consumed in the final growth stages of the plant. Wheatgrass however, comes from the early stages of growth from the wheat plant.

1920 - early 1930s - Dr. Charles Schnable - a food chemist - was looking for blood-building factors. His search was initiated while trying to reduce chicken death rates and improve laying hen's production of eggs.

What Dr. Schnable discovered was that the structure of an animal's blood (hemoglobin) was very similar to that of a plant's blood (chlorophyll) - the inner molecule in chlorophyll being magnesium, and in blood, it's iron.

Dr. Schnable conducted many experiments to find the blood-building factors, using a variety of vegetables, but mainly green vegetables, including grasses. He found the chickens were getting alfalfa in their feed, but when he increased alfalfa above 10% it became harmful to the animals. When he finally administered a mix of young wheatgrass and oatgrass, he hit pay dirt. The hen's winter laying production went from 38% on average to 94% and the eggshells were stronger too. Chickens fed this mix lacked the normal degenerative diseases that were commonly found in the production of chickens.

1930s- 1940s - Due to the Great Depression and World Wars, Americans suffered from the high cost and unavailability of fresh vegetables and dairy foods. A dehydrated form of grass was made available and widely used. This cereal grass product was comprised of Wheatgrass, oat and barley grass - known as cerophyl. The temperatures in which the grass leaves were dried, were as follows: for the first sixty seconds in excess of 1000°F. and after 60 seconds the temperatures were reduced to approximately 248°F. At these temperatures, all the enzymes should be dead as well as some vitamins. Yet, this grass still had a nutrient level exceeding other forms of food at that time.

By this time, the young stage of grass was presented officially as a food, given the high nutrient values for protein, minerals and vitamins. Additionally, it was discovered that the grass juice factor affected growth and couldn't be matched by substitution of vitamins A; B1, B2, B6 and D. the "Grass Juice Factor" won hands down.

Dr. Schnable was so impressed with these results that he personally integrated wheatgrass in his family's diet, who remained healthy with no serious illness or teeth problems as reported in the June 1st, 1942 article, "Fed His Family Grass for Eleven Years" in the Buffalo Courier Express.

During the 1940s, further research showed enhanced lactation (milk production) and reproduction ability in dairy cows, rabbits and rats following the 1930s studies on increased egg production in laying hens.

The impressive health benefits of Wheatgrass include:

Anti-cancer properties of Wheatgrass
Beginning in the early 1950s, studies showed how green vegetables, rich in chlorophyll, can furnish protection and even reduce damage caused by radiation treatments. The darker the green vegetable, the greater the reduction of damage caused by radiation.

Dr. Ernest Krells, the famous researcher of laetrile (an anticancer nutrient) claims that young Wheatgrass has ten times the laetrile than the seeds from which they sprout. There is research that shows Wheatgrass produces anti-cancer effects as well.

Plant extracts that are dark green and rich in chlorophyll, such as Wheatgrass juice extract, give protection from toxic chemicals and cancer-causing substances.

Note on colon cancer: Diets high in red meat and low in green vegetables are associated with increased colon cancer risk. Colon cancer is one of the leading causes of death from cancer in western societies.

Many epidemiological (a branch of medicine that deals in the prevalence of disease in large populations and detects the source and cause of epidemics of infectious diseases) studies have indicated that raw - and especially green - vegetables protect against colon cancer.

Note on liver cancer: According to Dr. Patricia A. Egner and colleagues, from Johns Hopkins University in Baltimore, Maryland, "…supplementation of diets with foods rich in chlorophyll may represent practical means to prevent the development of (liver cancer) or other environmentally induced cancers. It's an effective approach to chemo prevention and even simpler to implement in many regions of the world."

Note on prostate cancer: Researchers at the Fred Hutchinson Cancer Research Center conducted a study of 628 men ages 40 to 64 diagnosed with prostate cancer. Six hundred and two men of the same age without prostate cancer - found that men who consumed 28 or more servings of vegetables per week were found to have a 35% lower risk of prostate cancer than men who consumed fewer than 14 servings per week. It is believed that enzymes are activated by the different nutrients in vegetables and those help weaken cancer-causing substances found in the body.

Note on pancreatic cancer: A five-year study showed that consumption of dark leafy vegetables - along with onions, garlic, yellow vegetables, broccoli, and cauliflower - were found to be the vegetables most strongly associated with increased protection against pancreatic cancer.

The study, done at UCSF, University of California-San Francisco and supported by the National Cancer Institute, was one of the largest studies of its kind. Researchers Elizabeth A. Holly, PhD., June M. Chan, ScD and Furong Wang, M.D. found approximately a 50% reduction in developing pancreatic cancer by eating at least 5-9 servings per day of the above vegetables listed above. Fruit was found to be less protective than vegetables.

Note on breast cancer: Eydie Mae Hunsberger, a breast cancer survivor, wrote about using wheat grass juice as a component in her book "How I Conquered Cancer Naturally", Avery Publishers, 1992.

Note on skin cancer: Over an 11-year period, at the Queensland Institute, with over 1,000 Australian adults, showed a 41% decreased risk of skin cancer by increased amounts of dark green leafy vegetables. It also showed a 55% decrease in people who previously had skin cancer. This study was published in the International Journal of Cancer.

Eye Health
Other anti-oxidants - including lutein and zeaxanthin - found in Wheatgrass juice and other green vegetables are known to help prevent degenerative eye diseases, including cataracts and macular degeneration.

Chlorophyll: is the important factor in Wheatgrass juice and green vegetables.

Chlorophyll is a complex substance made up of carbon, hydrogen, magnesium, nitrogen and oxygen. The structure of these elements almost mirrors that of hemoglobin, the substance in human blood, which is the carrier of oxygen to cells throughout the body. Many nutrients are necessary for healthy blood and many of these nutrients are found in chlorophyll-rich foods such as wheatgrass.

Chlorophyll, found in all green foods, provides the most effective anti-mutagenic (against mutation cells) substance, which has been identified to date. In addition to chlorophyll, scientists have also identified many other constituents in plant life that they consider cancer preventing, such as bioflavonoids, folic acid, lutein, lycopene, sulforaphane -- all found in Wheatgrass juice.

Colon health and enemas

Plants pickup their nutrients from their root system. The health of the root system depends on its soil. Our intestinal tract is our "root system". Wheatgrass has an enormous root system that "digests" the elements in the soil and water and converts them to enzymes, anti-oxidants, mineral and vitamins. A study specific to digestive health was done with wheatgrass juice. This study was done on patients with ulcerative colitis. Symptoms and the disease were reduced.

Dr. Ann Wigmore (aka "the first lady of Wheatgrass") holistic health practitioner, nutritionist, and whole foods advocate, wrote in her book, The Hippocrates Diet and Health Program: "The use of wheatgrass juice in enema water or as a wheatgrass implant, has an even more powerful action on the colon muscles than plain water. The high magnesium content of the wheatgrass juice is in my opinion safer than coffee enemas used by many health clinics because wheatgrass doesn't introduce unwanted caffeine into the body."

The primary action of a retention enema is to clean up the toxins in the liver and has a smaller effect on cleansing the colon. Because toxins are circulating in our bloodstream, from a dirty liver and colon, cleansing these organs results in healthier cells, tissues and organs.

Age-defying Benefits
Healthy glowing skin is a reflection of our clean, strong, well-nourished root system and blood. Dr. Nicholas Perricone, in his book, "The Perricone Promise", Chapter 4, "Ten Superfoods for Age-Defying Beauty", recommends Wheatgrass juice for helping cholesterol, blood pressure, and immune response as well as being good for anti-aging and beauty.

Wheatgrass juice for the health of your blood and heart
Dr. Bernard Jensen, researcher, clinician and author of over 20 books on natural health, said, "Wheatgrass juice is one of the finest blood builders and body rejuvenators I know."

Dr. R.K. Marwaha at the Advanced Pediatric Centre, Postgraduate Institute of Medical Education and Research conducted a study over a 3-year period from 2000-2003. This study was done with Thalassemia patients. Thalassemia is a complex series of inherited disorders, which involve the molecule in red blood cells called hemoglobin which is responsible for carrying oxygen, being under-produced or absent. The end result is a most severe form of anemia. Fatigue, shortness of breath, bone deformities in the face as well as enlarged spleen, growth failure and poor appetite can result. Blood transfusions every 2-3 weeks are needed. If not treated, death results in 3-5 years. Marwaha is quoted as stating, "Wheatgrass juice has the potential to lower transfusion requirements in Thalassemics."

Beware – know where your vegetables come from
Here's how to be sure your vegetables have value: 1. Either grow your own vegetables (which in reality – most of us don't have the time). 2. Buy organic grown from nutrient rich soil. The soil in which your vegetables are grown is a vital key. These plants get their nourishment from the soil and pass on the quality and quantity of nutrients in which they're fed.

NOTE: The difference between "wheat grass" and Wheatgrass
The grass of the wheat plant grown in containers or trays at home or in a greenhouse has this spelling: "wheat grass". Wheatgrass grown outdoors in fields has this spelling: "Wheatgrass". Both are dark-green leafy vegetables.

My recommendation: Sweet Wheat®

Kim Bright, celebrated nutritionist and founder of Sweet Wheat, Inc., first discovered wheatgrass juice in 1977.

Bright spent eight years researching and farming Wheatgrass and discovered she could produce better nutrient values when the Wheatgrass was grown outside in nutrient-rich soil. The Wheatgrass grown outdoors could reproduce itself, in the mature stage, as wheat kernels. The homegrown tray style used in juice bars and greenhouses could not.

The stage at which harvest takes place is a big factor in how much nutrient value the Wheatgrass juice contains and is only present for a few days. At this time, the enzymes, proteins, minerals and vitamins are at their optimum nutrient delivery. At this point, (when the plant is preparing to create the new seed) known as " jointing stage." Now, it's wheat grass harvest time. The juice harvested at this stage will have all these nutrients the plant intended for its seed formation. At this perfect stage, the Wheatgrass has **No Gluten**.

That's why Sweet Wheat® wheatgrass is juiced and then freeze-dried. The wheatgrass juice is ten to twenty times more powerful as a nutrient supply than the cellulose-laden Wheatgrass. Sweet Wheat®'s organic wheatgrass juice powder is a good source of active enzymes, thus aiding even more the bioavailability of the nutrients because of its special harvesting.

Sweet Wheat® is taken 1-2 capsules or ½ - 1 gram daily servings. It is 10-20 times more concentrated and assimilates the juice immediately.

The difference:

Sweet Wheat® is certified Organic/Kosher, freeze-dried pure Wheatgrass juice powder. **Concentrated 10-20X more than just the Wheatgrass alone.** It comes in powder or in vegetable capsules and is gluten free. No fillers, binders or sweeteners are used - unlike some that have added arrowroot, maltodextrin or simply ground-up dried grass, fiber and all. These additives take away 20-80% of the nutrient value you would get in using just the juice.

If you choose to grow your own wheatgrass and juice it fresh be sure to buy a juicer specially made for Wheatgrass. And remember the better your soil, the better and more nutrient rich your wheatgrass will be. But if you're stretched for time and searching for convenience, superior quality, organic Wheatgrass juice loaded with bioactive, easily assimilated enzymes, minerals, vitamins and protein, then Sweet Wheat® is your best answer.

CHAPTER TWENTY

Whey Protein

So you want to be a *Superman (or woman)?*
The not-so-awful truth about Proteins

Faster than a speeding bullet, more powerful than a locomotive, and able to leap tall buildings in a single bound. Look, up in the sky—it's Superman!

If the legendary "Superman" had been a real person, what would you guess his secret was for his incredible stamina, amazing strength and incredibly good health? A reasonably educated guess: Whey Protein, also known as the "Gold Standard of Protein," one of the truly vital ingredients for a "super" diet.

Why is protein essential to our bodies?
The word protein comes from the Greek word "prota," which means "of primary importance." That's right. It's imperative to nurture our bodies every single day with protein.

Protein consists of essential and non-essential amino acids, giving us the foundation we absolutely need to keep our strength and our health. Here's why these non-essential and essential amino acids are so important: The body produces non-essential amino acids from other amino acids. Unfortunately, our bodies don't have the capacity to produce amino acids on their own. The only way to get the proper essential amino acids we need is by eating high-quality protein foods. We need protein to keep our body operating at maximum capacity so - it can:
- Repair body cells.
- Build and repair our muscles and bones.
- Keep our stamina and energy levels high.
- Maintain the processes in our body to keep our metabolism operating at peak performance.

What's the best source of protein?

Whey. (Even dedicated whey-lovers may not know the composition of whey. It's the refined liquid that remains after milk has been curdled and strained, a "cousin" or byproduct of cheese.)

Super protein for super powers
X-ray vision and the power to leap tall buildings like Superman may be promising a bit too much. But you'll be well on the way, mentally and physically. The magic of whey protein is that it feeds your brain, builds

stronger, bigger muscles, takes off fat and inches, prevents bone loss, and satisfies your hunger … like no other protein in the world.

Careful, now. Not all proteins are created equal. Here's how to compare:
- Quantity of amino acids;
- Rate of digestion and absorption;
- Fat content;
- Purity and taste.

Whey Protein: The muscle replenisher

Whey is truly the most soluble and easily digested protein you can put into your body. It's referred to as the "fast" protein because of its immediate ability to give on-the-spot nourishment to your muscles – and yes, that includes your heart and your brain. Not only does it contain all the essential amino acids; better yet, it contains an abundance of the amino acid leucine as well. (Leucine helps muscle growth and also keeps muscle tissue from degenerating).

It's all here. Whey contains more nourishment than any other protein, including milk, eggs and soy proteins. Dr. Donald Layman, professor at the University of Illinois, discovered that people who eat diets higher in the amino acid leucine have more lean muscle mass and less body fat, compared to those whose diet contain lower levels of leucine.

More important, whey is an excellent protein source for people of all ages who value the role a healthy diet plays in improving overall health. And because whey is a complete protein, it contains all the essential amino acids we need in our daily diets.

Now, who wouldn't want to ensure they get the greatest advantage to keep the body vital? There's more to be excited about:

The key to replenishing, repairing and rebuilding our muscles

Whey Protein is considered the "Gold Standard" of protein by those who use it and here's why: More than any other protein food source, whey protein contains the highest levels of branched chain amino acids (BCAAs). In addition to leucine, whey has isoleucine, needed for the formation of hemoglobin as well as assisting the regulation of blood sugar levels as well as energy levels. Whey too, contains valine, valuable for muscle metabolism, repair and growth of tissue and maintaining the nitrogen balance in the body.

Muscle repair is an important benefit because BCAAs activate the key enzymes in the protein that regenerate your muscles after physical exercise. During exercise or resistance training, BCAAs are metabolized directly into your muscle tissue. Considering this, whey is the only whole protein that can make the double claim to replenish depleted levels of BCAAs and repair and rebuild lean muscle tissue because of its high levels of BCAAs.

Where does whey protein come from?

What is the complex milk-derivative known as whey? It's made up of protein, minerals and trace amounts of fats. Of course protein is the most abundant ingredient in whey. The proteins found in milk are casein and whey. Of the two, whey protein is much more digestible than casein and represents a greater, higher caliber of protein that contains little or no fat. (Casein has its benefits, too. As a salt, it prevents "denaturing" – an assurance of ongoing strength in whey.)

Whey maintains a healthy immune system

When we exercise or resistance-train, our glutathione levels are reduced as well as the BCAAs. Glutathione is a tri-peptide of the amino acids cysteine, glycine, and glutamic acid. (Remember, our bodies can't produce amino acids on their own.) Glutathione is important because it's the master antioxidant of the body. Without glutathione, we can die. That's why it's crucial to constantly replenish our glutathione levels to boost our immune system. Whey helps our immune systems by increasing levels of glutathione in the body and giving us the essential amino acids to do this.

The foolproof step-by-step guide to becoming your own superman ... or woman

High protein diets have been found to reduce body weight and increase insulin sensitivity. What this means: Insulin concentration is associated with improved blood sugar control and reduced fat storage. So increasing dietary density with whey protein leads to a trimmer body ... which in turn means reduced weight gain.

Step #1: Maintain healthy weight without starving your brain or your body

Want to add healthy years to your life? Want to take the first step toward preventing weight related complications such as diabetes, cancer, and heart disease? We've all heard it before, but diet (the food we put in our bodies) really does play the main role in any weight management program.

As the rest of the world points out to us every day, eating is America's favorite national pastime. Whether you want to maintain a healthy weight, or would like to take off a few pounds while staying healthy and toned at the same time, the first step is to start your day with protein. Whey protein satisfies hunger, boosts your brainpower, and gets rid of food cravings as well. Here's why:

1. The body requires more energy to digest protein than it does to digest other foods. Result: You burn more calories after a protein meal.
2. Whey protein is pure protein with little to no fat or carbohydrates. It's a perfect complement to any low carbohydrate or low glycemic diet.
3. Whey protein contains the bioactive components to stimulate the release of two appetite-suppressing hormones, which are released into the system after eating. To support this, a new study found that whey protein had a greater impact on satiety than the other protein in milk, casein.

A nasty common effect of poor dieting is starvation (which affects us faster than we imagine): The self-imposed regiment of poor diet habits begins by starving our brains. Yes, our brains, and here's how the vicious cycle begins:

We have different types of neurotransmitters in our brain. One is the neurotransmitter called serotonin. If we have low levels of this neurotransmitter it not only affects our moods, anxiety, appetites, but we can even be prone to severe depression. Healthy levels of serotonin ensure we're relaxed, calm, and have the ability to cope with stress throughout our day. What often happens is we end up on anti-depressants because we don't know that lack of protein in our diet that can be the main reason for the depression.

Recommendation: Easy changes/big benefits.
Consider this: At the beginning of our day, most of us ingest sugar for breakfast (that includes hidden sugars) if we eat breakfast at all, feeding us a depressing day wrapped with anxiety and tension. Recommendation: To combat these effects and begin the day on a positive note, try feeding your brain, and stop your hunger pangs by adding whey protein to your breakfast menu.

The research backs it up.
Taking whey protein before meals helps eliminate hunger and food intake. Before you exercise, whey enhances the fat-burning effects of your workout. In essence, whey reduces hunger and caloric intake, promotes fat burning, and boosts the power to develop lean body mass.

Whey is the protein choice for all age groups who value maintaining and improving their health. Prediction: You'll feel more vital and actually see the difference in your skin, muscles, nails and all your body tissues.

> **Note for diabetics:** Whey helps reduce hunger and stops the necessity to produce insulin, making whey protein an excellent meal replacement for diabetics.

Step #2: Get up and move - it adds muscle and burns fat.

Our society, with all its perks and technology, has turned the average person into a "couch potato." Our lives have become sedentary.

Start recovery slowly with a regimen of exercise - you don't have win a marathon – but anything from walking, running, cycling, swimming or lifting weights add muscle and burn fat. Whey before and after your exercise ensures more efficiency through out the day.

Here's why: Your body requires protein before exercise to help burn fat and improve muscle mass. And two more important factors to consider, to take whey after your workout:

1. Protein helps repair muscles.
2. Protein gives your body a chance to lose fatty weight (rather than muscle weight).

After exercising, the body is hungry to replenish nutrients we've used; we have a two-hour opportunity to help our muscles grow – so the importance of feeding our muscles is vital during this time. Whey is an exceptional food source to get this done efficiently.

Here are some of the most apparent benefits whey has for endurance and strength:

1. Whey proteins are easily digestible (more so that meat).
2. The amino acids found in whey provide an energy source crucial for endurance exercise   and training.
3. Whey increases the release of growth hormone, which stimulates muscle growth.
4. Whey's bioactive compounds help improve immuno-function and gastrointestinal health.
5. Whey reduces excess free radical production in athletes when intensive exercise compromises the systems.

Step #3: Whey keeps the healthy pump of your heart

> **Heart Fact:** Heart disease kills one person every 34 seconds and is the leading cause of death in the United States for men and women alike.

Hypertension (high blood pressure) is one of the main leading causes of heart disease and stroke. Research proves that whey protein battles against hypertension. Clinical studies found that Whey helps reduce the blood pressure of borderline hypertensive individuals. Whey also promises to reduce elevated cholesterol.

Here's how whey protein works on the heart: Whey contains bioactive components that positively affect cardiovascular health. Whey-derived peptides protect against hypertension, inhibit platelet aggregation (clumping together of platelets in the blood), and lower blood cholesterol levels. These whey-bioactive components inhibit activity of angiotensin converting enzyme (ACE), the constrictor of vascular smooth muscle, which in turn, increases blood pressure. A number of whey protein-derived ACE inhibitors have been identified in a recent study in humans, showing that a specific Whey Protein Isolate with bioactive peptides reduced blood pressure in untreated borderline hypertensive adults after six weeks. Whey may also affect blood coagulation.

Step #4: The advantage of whey protein for cancer patients

Chemotherapy and radiation treatments not only kill the cancer but unfortunately also rob us of the nutritional requirements our bodies need to function. The results of chemotherapy and radiation on the body can be weight loss, muscle loss, and protein calorie malnutrition. And just like athletes, the glutathione levels become dangerously low during treatment, severely compromising the immune system. Whey Protein, rich in the amino acid cysteine, raises glutathione levels, reducing the risk of infection and improving the responsiveness to the immune system.

Evidence of anti-cancer activity

Unbelievable – cellular and animal studies indicate that whey and its peptides, as well as other components, may actually protect against some cancers as well. Laboratory animals given a diet that included whey showed promising results of reducing intestinal, breast, and colon cancers.

Two of the proteins in whey, administered orally in the post-initiation stage of the cancer, show that whey may inhibit colon, esophagus, lung, and bladder cancers as well.

Step #5: Fend off the risk of diabetes

Type II diabetes is a concern for everyone. How it's contracted isn't quite known, but one of the factors is obesity and high glucose levels. Type-2 diabetes is not unique to adults. It's becoming a major concern for children and teenagers as well. The good news is that you can help prevent and manage type II Diabetes by practicing healthy nutrition. Whey protein plays an important role in healthy nutrition and is an excellent choice for diabetics who need to carefully manage their food intake. Whey helps control blood glucose levels and weight and provides more value than equal amounts of lower quality proteins that are often higher in fat and cholesterol.

Step #6: Give your child a healthy start on life

Amazingly, whey is one of the key ingredients in baby formulas – including those formulas for premature infants. Of course, breast-feeding is the preferred choice for feeding your baby. Infant formulas containing Whey Protein are the next best thing if breast-feeding isn't an option.

Whey protein is an excellent choice during pregnancy as well, because increased amounts of protein is vitally essential. Pregnancy increases the body's protein needs by 33%. The expectant mother should consult with her doctor to determine her individual protein needs.

Baby note: Whey-based baby formulas have even been shown to reduce crying in colicky babies.

Step #7: Get the jump on heathly aging

By the year 2020 one of six Americans will be 65 and older. So bear in mind, muscle loss and its negative implications is becoming a big concern in terms of volume and medical costs. Good nutrition and adequate amounts of high quality protein along with exercise and resistance training help maintain strong muscles while we age.

Know the facts on aging:

- A recent study in Europe comparing whey protein to casein found that older men who consumed whey protein showed higher protein synthesis, helping to limit muscle loss over time.
- Whey protein also helps prevent bone loss. Another study at Boston University showed that older individuals who consumed low levels of protein had a significant loss of bone density, especially in the hips and spine.

Step #8: Guard against viruses

You can't discount protein for protection against toxins, bacteria, and viruses. Whey in particular contains several components such as immunoglobulins, lactoferrin and its peptide derivative, lactoferricin, are known to have antimicrobial and antiviral effects.

Whey Protein: Your insurance for outstanding healthy nutrition

In summary: The bioactive components in whey can protect against infections and viruses, enhance the immune system, protect against some cancers, and improve cardiovascular health -- not to mention the advantages for the physically active person.

As we become more knowledgeable about the potential health benefits of whey and its components, we're finding that its use in a variety of functional foods can be tailored to meet the health concerns of specific population groups.

What form of whey protein should you get? You can get whey protein in two different ways, Whey Isolate or Whey Concentrate. (Whey Isolate is the more pure and concentrated of the two. It contains 90% or more protein and little if any fat and lactose.) Whey Concentrate can have anywhere from 29 -89% protein depending on the product.

Nutritionists across the board recommend that you keep a variety of nutritious foods in your diet. To boost your body's ability to maintain its strength, health and balance, be sure to keep whey protein at the top of the list.

References

References

Aequorin

1. Adams, R.D., and M. Victor. Principles of Neurology. New York: McGraw-Hill Book Company, 1985.
2. Alexianu, M. et al. (1994). The role of calcium-binding proteins in selective motoneuron vulnerability in ALS. Annals of Neurology 36(6):846-858.
3. Appel, S.H. (1993). Excitotoxic neuronal cell death in ALS. Trends in Neuroscience 16: 3-5.
4. Baimbridge, K. et al. (1992). Calcium-binding proteins in the nervous system. Trends in Neuroscience 15(8):303-308.
5. Blinks, J. (1990). Use of photoproteins as intracellular calcium indicators. Environmental Health Perspectives 83:75-81.
6. Detert, J.A. et al. (2006). Neuroprotective effects of aequorin on hippocampal CA1 neurons following ischemia. Scientific abstract, Neuroscience.
7. Disterhoft, J.F., R.J. Moyer, and L.T. Thompson (1994).The calcium rationale in aging and Alzheimer's disease. Evidence from an animal model of normal aging. Annals of the New York Academy of Sciences 747:382-406.
8. Duncan, C. (1987). Role of intracellular calcium in promoting muscle damage: a strategy for controlling the dystrophic condition. Experientia 34:1531-1535.
9. Duthie, G.G. and J.R. Arthur. (1993). Free radicals and calcium homeostasis: relevance to malignant hyperthermia? Free Radical Biology and Medicine 14(4):435-442.
10. Eisen, A. (1995). ALS is a multifactorial disease. Muscle-Nerve 18(7):741-752.
11. Fleckenstein-Grun, G. and A. Fleckenstein (1991). Calcium—a neglected key factor in arteriosclerosis. The pathogenic role of arterial calcium overload and its prevention by calcium antagonists. Annals of Medicine 23(5):589-599.
12. Gibson, G. and C. Peterson (1987). Calcium and the aging nervous system. Neurobiology Aging 8:329-343.
13. Halliwell, B. (1989). Oxidants and the central nervous system: some fundamental questions. Acta Neural Scandinavia 126:23.
14. Hartmann et al. (1994). Disturbances of the neuronal calcium homeostasis in the aging nervous system. Life Science 55(25-26):2011-2018.
15. Heizmann, C. and K. Braun (1992). Changes in Ca(+2)-binding proteins in human neurodegenerative disorders. Trends in Neurosciences 15(8):259-264.
16. Iacopino, A., and S. Christakos (1990). Specific reduction of calcium-binding protein (28-kilodalton calbindin-D) gene expression in aging and neurodegenerative diseases. Proceedings of the National Academy of Sciences USA 87:4078-4082.
17. Iacopino, A., and S. Christakos (1984). Specific alterations in calcium-binding protein gene expression in neurodegenerative diseases. Abstract. UCLA Symposium of Neurodegenerative Diseases.
18. Ibarreta, D. et al. (1997). Altered Ca(2+) homeostasis in lymphoblasts from patients with late-onset Alzheimer's disease. Alzheimer Disease Association Disorders

11(4):220-227.

19. Ichmiya, Y. et al. (1988). Loss of calbindin-D28k immunoreactive neurons from the cortex in Alzheimer-type dementia. Brain Research 475:156.

20. Imbert, N. et al. (1995). Abnormal calcium homeostasis in DMD myotubes contracting in vitro. Cell Calcium 18:177-186.

21. Ince, P. et al. (1993). Parvalbumin and calbindin D28k in the human motor system and in motoneuron disease. Neuropathology Applied Neurobiology 19(4):291-299.

22. Inouye et al. (1985). Cloning and sequence analysis of DNA for the luminescent protein aequorin. Proceedings of the National Academy of Sciences USA 82:3154-3158.

23. Khachaturian, Z.S. (1994). Calcium hypothesis of Alzheimer's disease and brain aging. Annals of the New York Academy of Sciences 747:1-11.

24. Khachaturian, Z.S. (1989). Introduction and overview: calcium, membranes, aging and AD. Z.S. Khachaturian, C.W. Cotman, and J.W. Pettigrew, eds. Annals of the New York Academy of Sciences 568:1-4.

25. Lally, G. et al. (1997). Calcium homeostasis in aging: studies on the calcium binding protein calbindin D28k. Journal of Neural Transmission 104(10):1107-1112.

26. Lamm, Richard D. and Robert H. Blank. The challenge of an aging society. The Futurist, July-August, 2005.

27. Landfield, P.W. et al. (1992). Mechanisms of neuronal death in brain aging and AD: role of endocrine-mediated calcium dyshomeostasis. Journal of Neurobiology 23:1247-1260.

28. Leslie, S.W. et al. (1985). Reduced calcium uptake by brain mitochondria and synaptosomes in response to aging. Brain Research 329:177-183.

29. Lipton, S.A. and S.B. Kater (1989). Neurotransmitter regulation of neuronal outgrowth, plasticity, and survival. Trends in Neurological Sciences 12:265-270.

30. Mattson, M.P. (1992). Calcium as a sculptor and destroyer of neural circuitry. Experimental Gerontology 27:29-49.

31. Mattson, M.P. (1989). Cellular signaling mechanisms common to the development and degeneration of neuroarchitecture. Mechanisms of Ageing and Development 50:103-157.

32. Mattson, M.P. and B. Cheng. (1993). Growth factors protect neurons against excitotoxic/schemic damage by stabilizing calcium homeostasis. Stroke 24 (Supplement 1):36-40.

33. Mattson, M.P. et al. (2000). Calcium signaling in the ER: its role in neuronal plasticity and neurodegenerative disorders. Trends in Neurological Sciences 23(5):222-229.

34. McLachlan, D. et al. (1987). Calmodulin and calbindin D28k in Alzheimer's disease. Alzheimer Disease and Associated Disorders 1(3):171-179.

35. Meyer, F.B. (1989). Calcium, neuronal hyperexcitability and ischemic injury. Brain Research Brain Research Review 14(3):227-243.

36. Morrison, B.M. et al. (1998). Determinants of neuronal vulnerability in neurodegenerative diseases. Annals of Neurology 44:S32-S44.

37. Mouatt-Progent, A. et al. (1994). Does the calcium-binding protein calreticulin

protect dopaminergic neurons against degeneration in Parkinson's disease? Brain Research 668(1-2):62-70.

38. Moyer, J.R., Jr., S.M. Kelsey, J.P. McGann, and T.H. Brown (2001). Morphology and distribution of calbindin-D28k in adult and aged rat perirhinal cortex. Society for Neuroscience Abstracts 27, program number 327.7.

39. Moyer, J.R., Jr., J.M. Power, L.T. Thompson, and J.F. Disterhoft (2000). Increased excitability of aged rabbit CA1 neurons after trace eyeblink conditioning. Journal of Neuroscience 20:5476-5482.

40. Mukesh Chawla, Gordon Betcherman, and Arup Banerji. From Red to Gray: The Third Transition of Aging Populations in Eastern Europe and the Former Soviet Union. Washington, D.C.: World Bank, 2007.

41. Nixon, R. et al. (1994). Calcium-activated neutral proteinase (calpain) system in aging and AD. Annals of the New York Academy of Sciences 747:77-91.

42. Pascale, A. and Etcheberrigaray, R. (1999). Calcium alterations in Alzheimer's disease: pathophysiology models and therapeutic opportunities. Pharmacology Research 39(2): 81-88.

43. Rami, A., and J. Kriglstein. (1994). Neuronal protective effects of calcium antagonists in cerebral ischemia. Life Sciences 55(25-26):2105-2113.

44. Ripova, D. et al. (2004). Alterations in calcium homeostasis as a biological marker for mild Alzheimer's disease. Physiological Research 53:449-452.

45. Scharfman, H.E. and P.A. Schwartzkroin (1989). Protection of dentate hilar cells from prolonged stimulation by intracellular calcium chelation. Science 246:257-260.

46. Seto-Ohshima A., P.C. Emson, E. Lawson, C.Q. Mountjoy, and L.H. Carrasco (1988). Loss of matrix calcium-binding protein-containing neurons in Huntington's disease. Lancet 1(8597):1252-1255.

47. Shanahan, C. M. et al. (1994). High expression of genes for calcification-regulating proteins in human atherosclerotic plaques. Journal of Clinical Investigation 93(6):2393-2402.

48. Shaw, P. et al. (2000). Molecular factors underlying selective vulnerability of motoneurons to neurodegeneration in ALS. Journal of Neurology 247 (Supplement 1): 17-27.

49. Shimomura, O. A short story of aequorin. The Biological Bulletin, August 1, 1995.

50. Shimomura, O., F.H. Johnson, and Y. Saiga (1963). Further data on the bioluminescent protein, aequorin. Journal of Cellular and Comparative Physiology 62:1-8.

51. Shimomura, O., F.H. Johnson, and Y. Saiga (1962). Extraction, purification and properties of aequorin, a bioluminescent protein from the luminous hydromedusan, Aequorea. Journal of Cellular and Comparative Physiology 59:223-239.

52. Shimomura, O. and F.H. Johnson (1978). Peroxidized coelenterazine, the active group in the photoprotein aeqourin. Proceedings of the National Academy of Sciences USA 75: 2611-2615.

53. Shinichi, Iwasaki et al. (2000). Developmental changes in calcium channel types mediating central synaptic transmission. Journal of Neuroscience 20(1):59-65.

54. Siesjo, B.K. et al. (1989). Calcium, excitotoxins, and neuronaldeath in brain.

Annals of the New York Academy of Sciences 568:234-251.

55. Strazzullo, P. et al. (1986). Altered extracellular calcium homeostasis in essential hypertension: a consequence of abnormal cell calcium handling. Clinical Sciences 71(3): 239-246.

56. Sutherland, M. et al. (1993). Reduction of calbindin-28k mRNA levels in Alzheimer as compared to Huntington hippocampus. Brain Research Molecular Brain Research 18(1-2):32-42.

57. Underwood, M. The Aequorin Hypothesis—Calcium-Binding Proteins and Disease. A research monograph. Self-published, 1996.

58. Verity, M.A. (1992). Ca(2+)-dependent processes as mediators of neurotoxicity. Neurotoxicology 13:139-148

59. Yamada, T. et al. (1990). Relative sparing of Parkinson's disease of substantia nigra dopamine neurons containing calbindin D28k. Brain Research 526:303-307.

Andrographis paniculata

1. Efficacy and safety of an Andrographis paniculata formulation for the relief of signs and symptoms of Rheumatoid Arthritis: A Prospective Randomized Placebo-Controlled Trial.
Burgos1*, R.A., Hancke,1 J.L; Bertoglio2,3 J.C.; Cáceres4, D.D.; Aguirre5, V.; Arriagada6, S.; Calvo3 M.
1 Institute of Pharmacology, Faculty of Veterinary Sciences, Universidad Austral de Chile;
2 Unit of Immunology, Unit of Rheumatology and Unit of Critical Patients, Institute of Medicine, Faculty of Medicine, Universidad Austral de Chile, Hospital Regional de Valdivia, Chile;
3 Unit of Critical Patients, Institute of Medicine, Faculty of Medicine, Universidad Austral de Chile, Hospital Regional de Valdivia, Chile;
4 Division of Epidemiology, School of Public Health, Faculty of Medicine, Universidad de Chile, Santiago, Chile.
5 Unit of Rheumatology Institute of Medicine, Faculty of Medicine, Universidad Austral de Chile, Hospital Regional de Valdivia, Chile; Department of Medicine, Unit of Rheumatology, Hospital Regional de Osorno, Chile.

2. DOUBLE BLIND PLACEBO CONTROLLED STUDY ON THE EFFECT OF PARACTIN® ON RHEUMATOID ARTHRITIS. Verónica Aguirre MD, Rheumatologist1,2; Sonia Arriagada MD, Rheumatologist3; Juan C. Bertoglio MD, Clinical Immunologist1,2; Mario Calvo MD, Infectologist1,2; Rafael Burgos DVM, MSc, Pharmacologist4; Juan Hancke DVM, PhD4.; 1Faculty of Medicine, Universidad Austral de Chile, Valdivia Chile. Regional Hospital of Valdivia; Regional Hospital of Osorno; Institute of Pharmacology, Universidad Austral de Chile

3. ParActin® is useful for preventing memory loss in Alzheimer disease by activation of PPAR Receptor. Juan L. Hancke. Instituto de Farmacologia, Universidad Austral de Chile, Valdivia Chile.

4. Andrographolide interferes with T cell activation and reduces experimental

autoimmune encephalomyelitis in the mouse. MI, Tobar JA, Gonzalez PA, Sepulveda SE, Figueroa CA, Burgos RA, Hancke JL, Kalergis AM. Universidad Austral de Chile. Published: J Pharmacol Exp Ther. 2005 Jan;312(1):366-72. Epub 2004 Aug 26.

5. ParActin® interferes with DNA binding of NF-B in HL-60/Neutrophils cells. María A. Hidalgo, Alex Romero, Jaime Figueroa, Patricia Cortés, Ilona I. Concha, Juan L. Hancke, & Rafael A. Burgos. Uniersidad Austral de Chile. Published: British Journal of Pharmacology (2005) 144, 680-686

6. Andrographolide inhibits IFN and IL-2 cytokines production and protects against cell apoptosis 1Juan L. Hancke, & 1Rafael A. Burgos, Karina Seguel,Mirna Perez, Ada Meneses, Marcele Ortega. Published: Planta Med. 2005 May;71(5):429-34.

7. ParActin® EXHIBIT IMMUNOSTIMULANT EFFECT BY INCREASING CELLULAR INMUNE RESPONSE Juan L. Hancke, & 1Rafael A. Burgos

Carnosine

1. Aksenova MV, Aksenov MY, Markesbery WR, et al. Aging in a dish: age-dependent changes of neuronal survival, protein oxidation, and creatine kinase BB expression in long-term hippocampal cell culture. J Neurosci Res. 1999; 58(2):308-17.

2. Berlett BS, Stadtman ER. Protein oxidation in aging, disease, and oxidative stress. J Biol Chem. 1997; 272(33):20313-6.

3. Bierhaus A, Hofmann MA, Ziegler R, et al. AGEs and their interaction with AGE-receptors in vascular disease and diabetes mellitus. I. The AGE concept. Cardiovascular Research. 1998; 37(3):586-600.

4. Boldyrev A, Song R, Lawrence D, et al. Carnosine protects against excitotoxic cell death independently of effects on reactive oxygen species. Neuroscience. 1999; 94(2):571-7.

5. Boldyrev AA, Stvolinsky SL, Tyulina OV, et al. Biochemical and physiological evidence that carnosine is an endogenous neuroprotector against free radicals. Cell Mol Neurobiol. 1997; 17(2):259-71.

6. Brownson C, Hipkiss AR. Carnosine reacts with a glycated protein. Free Radic Biol Med. 2000; 28(10):1564-70.

7. Burcham PC, Kuhan YT. Diminished susceptibility to proteolysis after protein modification by the lipid peroxidation product malondialdehyde: inhibitory role for crosslinked and noncrosslinked adducted proteins. Arch Biochem Biophys. 1997; 340(2):331-7.

8. Butterfield DA. Alzheimer's b-amyloid peptide and free radical oxidative stress. Gilbert DL and Colton CA, editors. Reactive oxygen species in biological systems: an interdisciplinary approach. New York, 1999. Pp. 609-638.

9. Carney JM, Smith CD, Carney AM, et al. Aging- and oxygen-induced modifications in brain biochemistry and behavior. Ann NY Acad Sci. 1994; 738:44-53.

10. Carney JM, Starke-Reed PE, Oliver CN, et al. Reversal of age-related increase

in brain protein oxidation, decrease in enzyme activity, and loss in temporal and spatial memory by chronic administration of the spin-trapping compound N-tert-butyl-alpha phenylnitrone. Proc Natl Acad Sci USA. 1991; 88(9):3633-6.

11. Doble A. The role of excitotoxicity in neurodegenerative disease: implications for therapy. Pharmacol Ther. 1999; 81(3):163-221.

12. Forster MJ, Dubey A, Dawson KM, et al. Age-related losses of cognitive function and motor skills in mice are associated with oxidative protein damage in the brain. Proc Natl Acad Sci USA. 1996; 93(10):4765-9.

13. Gille JJ, Pasman P, van Berkel CG, et al. Effect of antioxidants on hyperoxia-induced chromosomal breakage in Chinese hamster ovary cells: protection by carnosine. Mutagenesis. 1991; 6(4):313-8.

14. Gulyaeva NV. Superoxide-scavenging activity of carnosine in the presence of copper and zinc ions. Biochemistry (Moscow). 1987; 52(7 Part 2):1051-4.

15. Gulyaeva NV, Dupin AM, Levshina IP. Carnosine prevents activation of free-radical lipid oxidation during stress. Bull Exp Biol Med. 1989; 107(2):148-152.

16. Hipkiss AR, Brownson C. A possible new role for the anti-ageing peptide carnosine. Cell Mol Life Sci. 2000; 57(5):747-53.

17. Hipkiss AR, Michaelis J, Syrris P. Non-enzymatic glycosylation of the dipeptide L-carnosine, a potential anti-protein-cross-linking agent. FEBS Lett. 1995; 371(1):81-5.

18. Hipkiss AR, Michaelis J, Syrris P, et al. Strategies for the extension of human life span. Perspect Hum Biol. 1995; 1:59-70.

19. Hipkiss AR, Preston JE, Himswoth DT, et al. Protective effects of carnosine against malondialdehyde-induced toxicity towards cultured rat brain endothelial cells. Neurosci Lett. 1997; 238(3):135-8.

20. Hipkiss AR, Preston JE, Himsworth DT, et al. Pluripotent protective effects of carnosine, a naturally occurring dipeptide. Ann NY Acad Sci. 1998; 854:37-53.

21. Horning MS, Blakemore LJ, Trombley PQ. Endogenous mechanisms of neuroprotection: role of zinc, copper, and carnosine. Brain Res. 2000; 852(1):56-61.

22. Kasai H. Analysis of a form of oxidative DNA damage, 8-hydroxy-2'-deoxyguanosine, as a marker of cellular oxidative stress during carcinogenesis. Mutat Res. 1997; 387(3):147-63.

23. McFarland GA, Holliday R. Retardation of the senescence of cultured human diploid fibroblasts by carnosine. Exp Cell Res 1994; 212(2):167-75.

24. McFarland GA, Holliday R. Further evidence for the rejuvenating effects of the dipeptide L-carnosine on cultured human diploid fibroblasts. Exp Gerontol. 1999; 34(1):35-45.

25. Mark RJ, Lovell MA, Markesbery WR, et al. A role for 4-hydroxynonenal, an aldehydic product of lipid peroxidation, in disruption of ion homeostasis and neuronal death induced by amyloid beta-peptide. J Neurochem. 1997; 68(1):255-64.

26. Munch G, Mayer S, Michaelis J, et al. Influence of advanced glycation end-products and AGE-inhibitors on nucleation-dependent polymerization of beta-amyloid peptide. Biochim Biophys Acta. 1997; 1360(1):17-29.

27. Munch G, Schinzel R, Loske C, et al. Alzheimer's disease--synergistic effects of glucose deficit, oxidative stress and advanced glycation endproducts. Journal of Neural Transmission. 1998; 105(4-5):439-61.

28. Nagai K, Suda T, Kawasaki K, et al. Action of carnosine and beta-alanine on wound healing. Surgery. 1986; 100(5):815-21.

29. Preston JE, Hipkiss AR, Himsworth DT, et al. Toxic effects of beta-amyloid(25-35) on immortalised rat brain endothelial cell: protection by carnosine, homocarnosine and beta-alanine. Neurosci Lett. 1998; 242(2):105-8.

30. Quinn PJ, Boldyrev AA, Formazuyk VE. Carnosine: its properties, functions and potential therapeutic applications. Mol Aspects Med. 1992; 13(5):379-444.

31. Stadtman ER. Protein oxidation and aging. Science. 1992; 257(5074):1220-4.

32. Stadtman ER, Levine RL. Protein oxidation. Ann NY Acad Sci. 2000; 899:191-208.

33. Stuerenburg HJ, Kunze K. Concentrations of free carnosine (a putative membrane-protective antioxidant) in human muscle biopsies and rat muscles. Arch Gerontol Geriatr. 1999. 29: 107-113.

34. Stvolinsky SL, Kukley ML, Dobrota D, et al. Carnosine: an endogenous neuroprotector in the ischemic brain. Cell Mol Neurobiol. 1999; 19(1):45-56.

35. Thomas T, Thomas G, McLendon C, et al. b-Amyloid-mediated vasoactivity and vascular endothelial damage. Nature. 1996; 380(6570):168-71.

36. Yan SD, Chen X, Fu J, et al. RAGE and amyloid-beta peptide neurotoxicity in Alzheimer's disease. Nature. 1996; 382(6593):685-91.

37. Yuneva MO, Bulygina ER, Gallant SC, et al. Effect of carnosine on age-induced changes in senescence-accelerated mice. J Anti-Aging Med. 1999; 2(4):337-42.

38. Zaloga GP, Roberts PR, Black KW. Carnosine is a novel peptide modulator of intracellular calcium and contractility in cardiac cells. Am J Physiol 1997; 272(1 Pt 2):H462-8.

Cell Oxygenation

1. Dyer, David S. Cellfood: Vital Cellular Nutrition for the New Millenium; A compelling report on a dietary supplement that is offering new hope for nutrient-starved human beings.

Colostrum

2. Ballard F, Wallace J, Francis G, Read L, Tomas F. (1996) Des (1-3) IGF-1: a truncated form of insulin-like growth factor-1. International Journal of Cellular Biology. 28:1085-1087.

3. Burrin D, Davis T, Ebner S, Schoknecht P, Fiorotto M, Reeds P. (1997) Colostrum enhances the nutritional stimulation of vital organ protein synthesis in neonatal pigs. American Society for Nutritional Sciences. 127(7):1284-9.

4. Cass TL. Insulin-like growth factor-1 (IGF-1, Somatomedin C) blood levels are not associated with prostate specific antigen (PSA) levels or prostate cancer: A study of 749 patients. Medical College of Wisconsin, Milwaukee, WI

5. Francis GL, Read LC, Ballard FJ, Bagley CJ, Upton FM, Gravestock PM, Wallace JC. (1986) Purification and partial sequence analysis of insulin-like growth factor-1 from bovine colostrum. Journal of Biochemistry 233:207-213.

6. Francis GL, Upton FM, Ballard FJ, McNeil KA, Wallace JC. (1988) Insulin-like growth factors 1 and 2 in bovine colostrum. Journal of Biochemistry. 251(1):95-103.

7. Juskevich J. (1990) Bovine Growth Hormone: Human Food Safety Evaluation. Science. 249(4971):875-83.

8. Armogida, SA, Yannaras, NM, Melton, AL, Srivastava, MD. (2004) Identification and quantification of innate immune system mediators in human breast milk. Allergy and Asthma Proceedings 25(5):297-304.

9. Bishop GA, Haxhinasto SA, Stunz LL, Hostager BS. (2003) Antigen-specific B-lymphocyte activation. Critical Reviews in Immunology 23(3):159-197.

10. Bitzan MM, Gold BD, Philpott DJ, Huesca M, Sherman PM, Karch H, Lissner R, Lingwood CA, Karmali MA. (1998) Inhibition of Helicobacter pylori and Helicobactor mustelae binding to lipid receptors by bovine colostrum. The Journal of Infectious Diseases 177(4):955-961.

11. Boesman-Finkelstein M. and Finkelstein R. (1989) Passive oral immunisation of children. Lancet 2(8675):1336.

12. Collins AM, Roberton DM, Hosking CS, Flannery GR. (1991) Bovine milk, including pasteurised milk, contains antibodies directed against allergens of clinical importance to man. International Archives of Allergy and Applied Immunology 96(4):362-7.

13. Ebina T, Sato A, Umezu K, Ishida N, Ohyama S, Ohizumi A, Aikawa K, Katagiri S, Katsushima N, Imai A. (1983) Prevention of rotavirus infection by cow colostrum containing antibody against human rotavirus. Lancet. 2(8357):1029-30.

14. Feldmann M, Brennan F, Maini R. (1996) Role of cytokines in rheumatoid arthritis. Annual Review of Immunology 14:397-440.

15. Feldmann M, Maini RN. (1999) The role of cytokines in the pathogenesis of rheumatoid arthritis. Rheumatology 38(suppl.2):3-7.

16. Huppertz H, Rutkowski S, Busch D, Eisebit R, Lissner R, Karch H. (1999) Bovine colostrum ameliorates diarrhea in infection with diarrheagenic Escherichia coli, shiga toxin producing E. coli, and E-coli expressing intimin and hemolysin. Journal of Pediatric Gastroenterology and Nutrition. 29(4):452-6.

17. Khazenson L, Gennad'eva T, Roshchin V, Krasheniuk A, Semenova N. (1980) Activity of bovine colostral IgG in the human digestive tract. Zhurnal Mikrobiologii, Epidemiologii, i Immunobiologii 9:101-6.

18. Loimaranta V, Carlen A, Olsson J, Tenovuo J, Syvaoja E.-L, Korhonen H. (1998) Concentrated bovine colostral whey proteins from Streptococcus mutans/Strep. sobrinus immunized cows inhibit the adherence of Strep. mutans and promote the aggregation of mutans streptococci. Journal of Dairy Research 65(4):599-607.

19. Mickelson KN, Moriarty KM. Immunoglobulin levels in human colostrum and milk. Journal of Pediatric Gastroenterology and Nutrition 1(3):381-4 (1982).

20. Milgrom H. (2002) Attainments in atopy: special aspects of allergy and IgE. Advances in Pediatrics 49:273-297.

21. Parodi PW. (1997) Cows' milk fat components as potential anticarcinogenic agents. Journal of Nutrition 127(6):1055-60.
22. Carver JD, Barness LA. Trophic factors for the gastrointestinal tract. Clinical Perinatology 23(2):265-285 (1996).
23. Crissinger K., Kvietys P. Granger D. (1990) Pathophysiology of gastrointestinal mucosal permeability. Journal of Internal Medicine Supplement 732:145-54.
24. Deitch E. (1990) The Role of intestinal barrier failure and bacterial translocation in the development of systemic infection and multiple organ failure. Archives of Surgery 125(3):403-4.
25. Doe W. (1979) An overview of intestinal immunity and malabsorption. American Journal of Medicine. 67(6):1077-84.
26. Galland, L. (1995, Aug/Sept) Leaky Gut Syndromes: Breaking the Vicious Cycles. Townsend Letter for Doctors 145:62.
27. Hollander D. (1999) Intestinal permeability, leaky gut, and intestinal disorders. Current Gastroenterology Reports 1(5):410-416.
28. Kim JW, Jeon WK, Yun JW, Park DI, Cho YK, Sung IK, Sohn CI, Kim BI, Yeom JS, Park HS, Kim EJ, Shin MS. (2005) Protective effects of bovine colostrum on non-steroidal anti-inflammatory drug induced intestinal damage in rats. Asia Pacific Journal of Clinical Nutrition 14(1):103-7.
29. Lonnerdal B. Nutritional and physiologic significance of human milk proteins. American Journal of Clinical Nutrition 77(6):1537S-1543S (2003).
30. Playford RJ, Floyd DN, Macdonald CE, Calnan DP, Adenekan RO, Johnson W, Goodlad RA, Marchbank T. (1999) Bovine colostrum is a health food supplement which prevents NSAID induced gut damage. Gut 44(5):653-8.
31. Playford RJ, MacDonald CE, Johnson WS. (2000) Colostrum and milk-derived peptide growth factors for the treatment of gastrointestinal disorders. American Journal of Clinical Nutrition 72(1):5-14.
32. Walker, WA. (1987) Pathophysiology of intestinal uptake and absorption of antigens in food allergy. Annals of Allergy 59(5 Pt 2):7-16.

Cordyceps

1. Koh, J. H., Kim, K. M., Kim, J. M., song, J. C. and Suh, H. J. (2003a) Antifatigue and Antistress Effect of the Hot-Water Fraction from Mycelia of Cordyceps sinensis. Biol Pharm Bull. 26 (5), 691-694.
2. Koh, J. H., Kim, J. M., Chang, U. J. and Suh, H. J. (2003b) Hypocholesterolemic effect of hot-water extract from mycelia of Cordyceps sinensis. Biol Pharm Bull. 26 (1), 84-87.
3. Lo, H. C., Tu, S. T., Lin, K. C. and Lin, S. C. (2004) The anti-hyperglycemic activity of the fruiting body of Cordyceps in diabetic rats induced by nicotinamide and streptozotcin. Life Sci. 74 (23), 2897-2908.
4. Parcell, A. C., smith, J. M., Schulthies, S. S., Myrer, J. W. and Fellingham, G. (2004) Cordyceps Sinensis (CordyMax Cs-4) supplementation does not improve endurance exercise performance. Int J Sport Nutr Exerc Metab. 36 (3), 504-509.
5. Shin, K. H., Lim, S. S., Lee, S., Lee, Y. S. Jung, S. H. and Cho, S. Y. (2003) Anti-

tumour and immuno-stimulating activities of the fruiting bodies of Paecilomyces japonica, a new type of Cordyceps spp. Phytother Res. 17 (7), 830-833.

6. Wang, Y. H., Ye, J., Li, C. L., cai, S. Q., Ishizaki, M. and Katada, M. (2004) An experimental study on anti-aging action of Cordyceps extract. Zhongguo Zhong Yao Za Zhi. 29 (8), 773-776.

7. Wang, B. J., Won, S. J., Yu, Z. R. and Su, C. L. (2005) Free radical scavenging and apoptotic effects of Cordyceps sinensis fractionated by supercritical carbon dioxide. Food Chem Toxicol. 43 (4), 543-552.

8. Yalin, W., Ishurd, O., Cuirong, S. and Yuanjiang, P. (2005) Structure analysis and antitumour activity of (1à3)-bea-d-glucans (cordyglucans) from the mycelia of Cordyceps sinensis. Planta Med. 71 (4), 381-384.

9. Yamaguchi, Y., kagota, S., nakamura, K., Shinozuka, K. and Kunitomo, M. (2000) Inhibitory effects of water extracts from fruiting bodies of cultured Cordyceps sinensis on raised serum lipid peroxide levels and aortic cholesterol deposition in atherosclerotic mice. Phytother Res. 14 (8), 650-652.

10. Zhang, W., Yang, J., Chen, J., Hou, Y. and Han, X. (2005) Immunomodulatory and antitumour effects of an exopolysaccharide fraction from cultivated Cordyceps sinensis (Chinese caterpillar fungus) on tumour-bearing mice. Biotechnol Appl Biochem. 42 (pt 1, 9-15.

Enzymes

1. Cutler, Dr. Ellen. Micro Miracles: Discover the Healing Power of Enzymes. Holtzbrink Publishers/ 2005.

2. Roitt I, Brostoff J, Male D. Cells involved in the immune response. In: Roitt I, Brostoff J, Male D (eds). Immunology. St. Louis, Mo: The CV Mosby Co; 1985: 2.1-2.16.

3. Desser, L., Rehberger, A., "Induction of tumor necrosis factor in human peripheral-blood mononuclear cells by proteolytic enzymes," Oncology 47:475-77 (1990).

4. Nutrition Science News, May 1997.

5. The Penguin Dictionary of Biology.

6. Oxford Dictionary of Biology.

Fish Oil

1. Lai L, et al. Generation of cloned transgenic pigs rich in omega-3 fatty acids. Nature Biotechnology 2006;24:435–436.

2. Emken EA, Adlof RO, Gulley RM. Dietary linoleic acid influences desaturation and acylation of deuterium-labeled linoleic and linolenic acids in young adult males. Biochim Biophys Acta 1994;1213:277–288.

3. Pawlosky RJ, Hibbeln JR, Novotny JA, et al. Physiological compartmental analysis of alpha-linolenic acid metabolism in adult humans. J Lipid Res 2001;42:1257–1265.

4. Marchello, MJ. Nutrient composition of grass and grain finished bison. Great Plains Research 2001;11:65–82.

5. Simopolous, AP. Essential Fatty Acids in health and chronic disease. Am J Clin Nutr 1999;70:560S–569S.

6. Lerman R. Essential Fatty Acids. Integrative Medicine 2006;5:34–44.

7. Lin DS, Connor WE, Wolf DP, et al. Unique lipids of primate spermatozoa: desmosterol and docosahexaenoic acid. J Lipid Res 1993;34:491–499.

8. Neuringer M, Connor WE, Lin DS, et al. Biochemical and functional effects of prenatal and postnatal omega 3 fatty acid deficiency on retina and brain in rhesus monkeys. Proc Natl Acad Sci USA 1986 ;83:4021–4025.

9. Serhan CN, Gotlinger K, Hong S, et al. Resolvins, docosatrienes, and neuroprotectins, novel omega-3-derived mediators, and their aspirin-triggered endogenous epimers: an overview of their protective roles in catabasis. Prostaglandins Other Lipid Mediat 2004;73:155–172.

10. Serhan CN. Novel omega-3-derived local mediators in anti-inflammation and resolution. Pharmacol Ther 2005;105:7–21.

11. Mishra A, Chaudhary A, Sethi S. Oxidized omega-3 fatty acids inhibit NF-kappaB activation via a PPARalpha-dependent pathway. Arterioscler Thromb Vasc Biol 2004;24:1621–1627.

12. Li H, Ruan XZ, Powis SH, et al. EPA and DHA reduce LPS-induced inflammation responses in HK-2 cells: evidence for a PPAR-gamma-dependent mechanism. Kidney Int 2005;67:867–874.

13. Iribarren C, Markovitz J, Jacobs D, et al. Dietary intake of n-3, n-6 fatty acids and fish: relationship with hostility in young adults—the CARDIA study. Eur J Clin Nutr 2004;58:24–31.

14. Karlsson M, Mårild S, Brandberg J, et al. Serum Phospholipid Fatty Acids, Adipose Tissue, and Metabolic Markers in Obese Adolescents. The North American Association for the Study of Obesity 2006:14;1931-1939.

15. Neschen S, Morino K, Dong J, et al. n-3 Fatty Acids Preserve Insulin Sensitivity In Vivo in a Peroxisome Proliferator-Activated Receptor-{alpha}-Dependent Manner. Diabetes 2007;56:1034–1041.

16. Weiss LA, Barrett-Connor E, von Mühlen D. Ratio of n-6 to n-3 fatty acids and bone mineral density in older adults: the Rancho Bernardo Study. Am J Clin Nut 2005;81:934-938.

17. Burns J, Dockery D, Neas L, et al. Low dietary nutrient intakes and respiratory health in adolescents. Chest 2007.

18. Boelsma E, Hendriks HFJ, Roza L. Nutritional skin care: health effects of micronutrients and fatty acids. Am J Clin Nut 2001;73:853–864.

19. Nicolas G Bazan. Cell survival matters: docosahexaenoic acid signaling, neuroprotection and photoreceptors. Trends Neurosci 2006.

20. Ross BM, McKenzie I, Glen I, Bennett CP. Increased levels of ethane, a non-invasive marker of n-3 fatty acid oxidation, in breath of children with attention deficit hyperactivity disorder. Nutr Neurosci 2003;6: 277–281.

21. Crowe FL, et al. Serum phospholipid n-3 long-chain polyunsaturated fatty acids and physical and mental health in a population-based survey of New Zealand

adolescents and adults. Am J Clin Nutr 2007;86:1278–1285.

22. Rabini RA, Moretti N, Staffolani R, et al. Reduced susceptibility to peroxidation of erythrocyte plasma membranes from centenarians. Exp Gerontol 2002;37:657–663.

23. Kris-Etherton PM, Harris WS, Appel LJ; American Heart Association. Nutrition Committee. Fish consumption, fish oil, omega-3 fatty acids, and cardiovascular disease. Circulation 2002 Nov 19;106:2747–2757.

24. von Schacky C, Harris WS. Cardiovascular benefits of omega-3 fatty acids. Cardiovasc Res 2007 Jan 15;73:310–315.

25. von Schacky C, Harris WS.Cardiovascular risk and the omega-3 index. J Cardiovasc Med (Hagerstown) 2007 Sep;8 Suppl 1:S46–S49.

26. Richardson AJ. Clinical trials of fatty acid treatment in ADHD, dyslexia, dyspraxia and the autistic spectrum. Prostaglandins Leukot Essent Fatty Acids 2004;70:383–390.

27. Nurk E, et al. Cognitive performance among the elderly and dietary fish intake: the Hordaland Health Study. Am J Clin Nutr 2007;86:1470–1478.

28. Maes M, Christophe A, Delanghe J, et al. Lowered omega3 polyunsaturated fatty acids in serum phospholipids and cholesteryl esters of depressed patients. Psychiatry Res 199922;85:275–291.

29. Hibbeln JR. Fish consumption and major depression. Lancet 1998;351:1213.

30. Noaghiul S, Hibbeln JR. Cross-national comparisons of seafood consumption and rates of bipolar disorders. Am J Psychiatry 2003;160:2222–2227.

31. Stevens LJ, Zentall SS, Abate ML, et al. Omega-3 fatty acids in boys with behavior, learning, and health problems. Physiol Behav 1996;59:915–20.

32. Antalis CJ, Stevens LJ, Campbell M, et al. Omega-3 fatty acid status in attention-deficit/hyperactivity disorder. Prostaglandins Leukot Essent Fatty Acids 2006;75:299–308.

33. Richardson AJ, Montgomery P. The Oxford-Durham study: a randomized, controlled trial of dietary supplementation with fatty acids in children with developmental coordination disorder. Pediatrics 2005;115:1360–1366.

34. Patrick L, Salik R. Benefits of Essential Fatty Acid Supplementation on Language and Learning Skills in Children with Autism and Asperger's Syndrome.

35. Freeman MP, Hibbeln JR, Wisner KL, et al. Omega-3 Fatty Acids: Evidence Basis for Treatment and Future Research in Psychiatry. J Clin Psychiatry 2006;67:1954–1967.

36. Goldberg RJ, Katz J. A meta-analysis of the analgesic effects of omega-3 polyunsaturated fatty acid supplementation for inflammatory joint pain. Pain 2007 May;129:210–223.

37. Maroon JC, Bost JW. Omega-3 Fatty acids (fish oil) as an anti-inflammatory: an alternative to nonsteroidal anti-inflammatory drugs for discogenic pain. Surgical Neurology 2006;65:326–331.

38. Calder PC. n-3 polyunsaturated fatty acids, inflammation, and inflammatory diseases. Am J Clin Nutr 2006;83:1505S–1519S.

39. van Houwelingen AC, Sørensen JD, Hornstra G, et al. Essential fatty acid status in neonates after fish-oil supplementation during late pregnancy. Br J Nutr 1995;74:723-731.

40. Francois CA, Connor SL, Bolewicz LC, Connor WE. Supplementing lactating women with flaxseed oil does not increase docosahexaenoic acid in their milk. Am J Clin Nutr 2003;77:226–233.

41. Saldeen P, Saldeen, T. Women and Omega-3 Fatty Acids. Obstet Gynecol Surv 2004;59:722–730.

42. Colombo J, Kannass KN, Shaddy DJ, et al. Maternal DHA and the development of attention in infancy and toddlerhood. Child Dev 2004;75:1254–1267.

43. Dunstan JA, Mori TA, Barden A, et al. Fish oil supplementation in pregnancy modifies neonatal allergen-specific immune responses and clinical outcomes in infants at high risk of atopy: a randomized, controlled trial. J Allergy Clin Immunol 2003;112:1178–1184.

44. Dunstan JA, Roper J, Mitoulas L, Hartmann PE, et al. The effect of supplementation with fish oil during pregnancy on breast milk immunoglobulin A, soluble CD14, cytokine levels and fatty acid composition. Clin Exp Allergy 2004;34:1237–1242.

45. Helland IB, Smith L, et al. Maternal supplementation with very-long-chain n-3 fatty acids during pregnancy and lactation augments children's IQ at 4 years of age. Pediatrics 2003;111:e39–44.

46. McNamara RK, Carlson SE. Role of omega-3 fatty acids in brain development and function: potential implications for the pathogenesis and prevention of psychopathology. Prostaglandins Leukot Essent Fatty Acids 2006;75:329–349.

47. Simopoulos AP, Leaf A., Salem N. Workshop on the essentiality of and recommended dietary intakes for Omega-6 and Omega-3 fatty acids: Conference Report. J Am Coll Nutr 1999;18:487–489.

48. Birch E, Garfield S, Castaneda Y, et al. Visual acuity and cognitive outcomes at 4 years of age in a double-blind, randomized trial of long-chain polyunsaturated fatty acid-supplemented infant formula. (Epub)

49. Miljanovi B, Trivedi KA, Dana MR, et al. Relation between dietary n-3 and n-6 fatty acids and clinically diagnosed dry eye syndrome in women. Am J Clin Nutr 2005;82:887–893.

50. SanGiovanni JP, Chew EY, Clemons TE, et al. Age-Related Eye Disease Study Research Group. The relationship of dietary lipid intake and age-related macular degeneration in a case-control study: AREDS Report No. 20. Arch Ophthalmol 2007;125:671–679.

51. Townend BS, Townend ME, Flood V, et al. Dietary macronutrient intake and five-year incident cataract: the blue mountains eye study. Am J Ophthalmol 2007;143:932–939.

52. Rotstein NP, Politi LE, German OL, et al. Protective effect of docosahexaenoic acid on oxidative stress-induced apoptosis of retina photoreceptors. Invest Ophthalmol Vis Sci 2003;44:2252–2259.

53. AHRQ - Evidence reports and summaries - Effects of Omega-3 fatty acids on cardiovascular disease.
Covington MB. Omega-3 fatty acids. Am Fam Physician 2004;70:133–140.

54. Lawson LD, Hughes BG. Human absorption of fish oil fatty acids as

triacylglycerols, free acids, or ethyl esters. Biochem Biophys Res Commun 1988;152:328–335.

55. Beckermann B, Beneke M, Seitz I. Comparative bioavailability of eicosapentaenoic acid and docasahexaenoic acid from triglycerides, free fatty acids and ethyl esters in volunteers. Arzneimittelforschung 1990;40:700–704.

56. Turner R, McLean CH, Silvers KM. Are the health benefits of fish oils limited by products of oxidation? Nutrition Research Reviews 2006;19:53–62.

57. Montine KS, Quinn JF, Zhang J, et al. Isoprostanes and related products of lipid peroxidation in neurodegenerative diseases. Chem Phys Lipids 2004;128:117–124.

58. U.S. Environmental Protection Agency WEBSITE: http://www.epa.gov/waterscience/fishadvice/advice.html.]

59. Melanson SF, et al. Measurement of organochlorines in commercial over-the-counter fish oil preparations: implications for dietary and therapeutic recommendations for omega-3 fatty acids and a review of the literature. Arch Pathol Lab Med 2005;129:74–77.

60. Foran SE, et al. Measurement of mercury levels in concentrated over-the-counter fish oil preparations: is fish oil healthier than fish? Arch Pathol Lab Med 2003;127:1603–1605.

GH3

1. Cohen S., Ditman K.S. Effects of erovital-H3 on Elderly Depressive Patients. Int. Smposium of Gerontology, Bucharest, 1972.

2. Teitel A., Gane P., Stroescu V., Steflea D., About the Mechanisms of Procaine. Studies of Fisiology, Bucharest, 1962, 4, 351-360.

3. Gordon P., Fudema A., Abrams A., Effects of Romanian and American Procaine Preparations on Certain Physiological Aspects of Aging. Gerontologist II, 1962, p.9, Gerontologist, 1965, 20, 2, p114-150.

4. Ana Aslan; Gerovital-H3 Therapy in the Prophylaxis of Ageing. Rom. J. Geront. Geriatrics. Bucharest, 1980, 1,1 p5-15.

5. Yau M.T. Gerovital-H3, Monoamineoxidase and Brain Monoamines. Symposium on Theoretic Aspects of Aging, 1974, Miami, Florida.

6. Parhon C.I., Ana Aslan, L'action de la Vitamine H1 et H2 sur la proliferation de la cellule animale. Bull. Acad. Rom. Bucharest, 1957, 9,1, 137.

7. Berger P; Innocuite du traitment chronique a la procaine chez le rat en croissance. C.R. So. Biol. 1960, 154,959.

8. Verzar F. Note on the influence of prcaine, PABA and DEAE on the aging of rats. Basel, 1959, Gerontology 3,6, 350-355.

9. Ana Aslan et col. Long term treatment with Gerovital-H3 in Albino rats. J. Gerontology, 1965, 20,1.

10. Ana Aslan, G. Enachescu. Reseaches on the Anti-thrombophilic activity of Gerovital-H3 treatment. Rom. J. Geront. Geriatrics, 180, 1, 2, 195-246.

11. Russu C et col. Antioxidant and lipid lowering effect of original procaine based product Gerovital-H3. Book of abstracts. The 16th Congress of the Internatonal

Association of Gerontology, p217.

12. Zung W.W.K., Wang H.S. Clinical trials of Gerovital-H3 in the treatment of depression in the elderly. 10th Int. Congress of Gerontology, 1975, Jerusalem.

13. McFarlane M.D. Gerovital-H3 therapy; Mechanism of inhibition ofmonoamineoxidase. J. of American Geriatrics Society., 1974, XXII/8, p365-371.

14. Robinson D.S. et al; Aging, monoamine and monoamineoxidase levels, 1972, Lancet, 1, 0290.

15. Luth P. Aslan therapie mit Gerovital-H3. Zeitschrift fur Algemenmedizin, 1984, 60, 27, p1162-1164.

Hyaluronic Acid

1. Mazieres B, Bannwarth B, Dougados M, Lequesne M. EULAR recommendations for the management of knee osteoarthritis: report of a taskforce of the Standing Committee for International Clinical Studies Including Therapeutic Trials. Joint Bone Spine. 2001;68:231-240.

2. Pendleton A, Arden N, Dougados M, et al. EULAR recommendations for the management of knee osteoarthritis: report of a taskforce of the Standing Committee for International Clinical Studies Including Therapeutic Trials (ESCISIT). Ann Rheum Dis. 2000;59:936-944.

3. Recommendations for the medical management of osteoarthritis of the hip and knee: 2000 update. American College of Rheumatology Subcommittee on Osteoarthritis Guidelines. Arthritis Rheum. 2000;43:1905-1915.

4. Felson DT, Anderson JJ. Hyaluronate sodium injections for osteoarthritis: hope, hype, and hard truths. Arch Intern Med. 2002;162:245-247.

5. Brandt KD, Smith GN Jr, Simon LS. Intraarticular injection of hyaluronan as treatment for knee osteoarthritis: what is the evidence? Arthritis Rheum. 2000;43:1192-1203.

6. Synvisc-Hylan G-F 20 [package insert]. Ridgefield, NJ: Biometrics Inc; 2000.

7. Altman R, Brandt K, Hochberg M, et al. Design and conduct of clinical trials in patients with osteoarthritis: recommendations from a taskforce of the Osteoarthritis Research Society: results from a workshop. Osteoarthritis Cartilage. 1996;4:217-243.

8. Cohen J. Statistical Power Analysis for the Behavioral Sciences. 2nd ed. Hillsdale, NJ: L Erlbaum Associates; 1988:xxi, 567.

9. Felson DT. The verdict favors nonsteroidal antiinflammatory drugs for treatment of osteoarthritis and a plea for more evidence on other treatments. Arthritis Rheum. 2001;44:1477-1180. Liang MH, Larson MG, Cullen KE, Schwartz JA. Comparative measurement efficiency and sensitivity of five health status instruments for arthritis research. Arthritis Rheum. 1985;28:542-547. ISI | PUBMED

10. Roos EM, Nilsdotter AK, Toksvig-Larsen S. Patient expectations suggest additional outcomes in total knee replacement [abstract]. Arthritis Rheum. 2002;46(suppl):9.

11. Dixon AS, Jacoby RK, Berry H, Hamilton EB. Clinical trial of intra-articular injection of sodium hyaluronate in patients with osteoarthritis of the knee. Curr Med Res Opin. 1988;11:205-213.

12. Russell IJ, Michalek JE, Lawrence VA, Lessard JA, Briggs BT, May GS. A randomized, placebo and no-intervention controlled, trial of intra-articular 1%

sodium hyaluronate in the treatment of knee osteoarthritis [abstract]. Arthritis Rheum. 1992;35(suppl):9.

13. Dougados M, Nguyen M, Listrat V, Amor B. High molecular weight sodium hyaluronate (hyalectin) in osteoarthritis of the knee: a 1 year placebo-controlled trial. Osteoarthritis Cartilage. 1993;1:97-103. 15. Puhl W, Bernau A, Greiling H. Intra-articular sodium hyaluronate in osteoarthritis of the knee: a multicenter, double-blind study. Osteoarthritis Cartilage. 1993;1:233-241.

14. Dahlberg L, Lohmander LS, Ryd L. Intraarticular injections of hyaluronan in patients with cartilage abnormalities and knee pain: a one-year double-blind, placebo-controlled study. Arthritis Rheum. 1994;37:521-528. ISI

15. Creamer P, Sharif M, George E, et al. Intra-articular hyaluronic acid in osteoarthritis of the knee: an investigation into mechanisms of action. Osteoarthritis Cartilage. 1994;2:133-140.

16. Henderson EB, Smith EC, Pegley F, Blake Dr. Intra-articular injections of 750 kD hyaluronan in the treatment of osteoarthritis: a randomised single centre double-blind placebo-controlled trial of 91 patients demonstrating lack of efficacy. Ann Rheum Dis. 1994;53:529-534.

17. Cohen MA, Shiroky JB, Ballechey ML, Neville C, Esdaile JM. Double-blind randomized trial of Intra-articular Hyaluronate in the treatment of osteoarthritis of the knee. Arthritis Rheum. 1994;34(suppl):6.

18. Scale D, Wobig M, Wolpert W. Viscosupplementation of osteoarthritic knees with hylan: a treatment schedule study. Curr Therapeut Res. 1994;55:220-232.

19. Corrado E, Peluso GF, Gigliotti S. The effects of intra-articular administration of hyaluronic acid on osteoarthritis of the knee: a clinical study with immunological and biochemical evaluations. Eur J Rheumatol Inflamm. 1995;15:47-56.

20. Sala SF, Miguel RE. Intra-articular hyaluronic acid in the treatment of osteoarthritis of the knee: a short-term study. Eur J Rheumatol Inflamm. 1995;15:33-38.

21. Carrabba M, Paresce E, Angelini M, Re KA, Torchiana EEM, Perbellini A. The safety and efficacy of different dose schedules of hyaluronic acid in the treatment of painful osteoarthritis of the knee with joint effusion. Eur J Rheumatol Inflamm. 1995;15:25-31.

22. Lohmander LS, Dalen N, Englund G, et al, for the Hyaluronan Multicentre Trial Group. Intra-articular hyaluronan injections in the treatment of osteoarthritis of the knee: a randomised, double blind, placebo controlled multicentre trial. Ann Rheum Dis. 1996;55:424-431. FREE FULL TEXT

23. Wobig M, Dickhut A, Maier R, Vetter G, et al. Viscosupplementation with hylan G-F 20: a 26-week controlled trial of efficacy and safety in the osteoarthritic knee. Clin Ther. 1998;20:410-423.

24. Altman RD, Moskowitz R, for the Hyalgan Study Group. Intraarticular sodium hyaluronate (Hyalgan) in the treatment of patients with osteoarthritis of the knee: a randomized clinical trial. J Rheumatol. 1998;25:2203-2212.

25. Huskisson EC, Donnelly S. Hyaluronic acid in the treatment of osteoarthritis of the knee. Rheumatology (Oxford). 1999;38:602-607.

26. Brandt KD, Block JA, Michalski JP, Moreland LW, Caldwell JR, Lavin PT, for the ORTHOVISC Study Group. Efficacy and safety of intraarticular sodium

hyaluronate in knee osteoarthritis. Clin Orthop. 2001;385:130-143.

27. Tamir E, Robinson D, Koren R, Agar G, Halperin N. Intra-articular hyaluronan injections for the treatment of osteoarthritis of the knee: a randomized, double-blind placebo controlled study. Clin Exp Rheumatol. 2001;19:265-270.

28. Petrella RJ, DiSilvestro MD, Hildebrand C. Effects of hyaluronate sodium on pain and physical functioning in osteoarthritis of the knee: a randomized, double-blind, placebo-controlled clinical trial. Arch Intern Med. 2002;162:292-298.

29. Karlsson J, Sjogren LS, Lohmander LS. Comparison of two hyaluronan drugs and placebo in patients with knee osteoarthritis: a controlled, randomized, double-blind, parallel-design multicentre study. Rheumatology (Oxford). 2002;41:1240-1248.

30. Pham T, Le Hananff A, Ravaud P. Lack of symptomatic and structural efficacy of a new hyaluroninc acid compound, (NRD101), when compared to diacerein and placebo in a one year controlled study in symptomatic knee osteoarthritis [abstract]. Artritis Rheum. 2003;48(suppl):9.

31. Jubb R, Piva S, Beinat L, Dacre I, Gishen P. A one-year, randomised, placebo (saline) controlled clinical trial of 500-730 kDa sodium hyaluronate (Hyalgan) on the radiological change in osteoarthritis of the knee. Int J Clin Pract. 2003;57:467-474.

32. Sterne JA, Gavaghan D, Egger M. Publication and related bias in meta-analysis: power of statistical tests and prevalence in the literature. J Clin Epidemiol. 2000;53:1119-1129.

33. Lexchin J, Bero LA, Djulbegovic B, Clark O. Pharmaceutical industry sponsorship and research outcome and quality: systematic review. BMJ. 2003;326:1167-1170.

34. Kirwan J. Is there a place for intra-articular hyaluronate in osteoarthritis of the knee? Knee. 2001;8:93-101.

35. Aviad AD, Houpt JB. The molecular weight of therapeutic hyaluronan (sodium hyaluronate): how significant is it? J Rheumatol. 1994;21:297-301.

36. Allard S, O'Regan M. The role of elastoviscosity in the efficacy of viscosupplementation for osteoarthritis of the knee: a comparison of hylan G-F 20 and a lower-molecular-weight hyaluronan. Clin Ther. 2000;22:792-795.

37. Block, A., and Bettelheim, F.: Water Vapor Sorption of Hyaluronic Acid, Biochim Biophys Acta 201, 69, 1970

38. Goa K. L. and Benfield P.: Drugs 1994, 47: 536-566.

39. Laurent, T., and Gergely, J.: Light Scattering Studies on Hyaluronic Acid, J Biol Chem 212, 325, 1955.

40. George E. Intra-articular hyaluronan treatment for osteoarthritis. Ann Rheum Dis 1998;57:637-40.

41. Wobig M, Bach G, Beks P, Dickhut A, Runzheimer J, Schwieger G, et al. The role of elastoviscosity in the efficacy of viscosupplementation for osteoarthritis of the knee: a comparison of hylan G-F 20 and a lower-molecular-weight hyaluronan. Clin Ther 1999;21:1549-62.

42. Weiss C, Balazs EA, St. Onge R, Denlinger JL. Clinical studies of the intraarticular injection of HealonR (sodium hyaluronate) in the treatment of osteoarthritis of human knees. Osteoarthritis symposium. Palm Aire, Fla., October 20-22, 1980. Semin Arthritis Rheum. 1981;11(suppl 1):143-4.

43. New Zealand Dermatological Society, Dec 2, 2002.

Lion's Mane

1. Kawagishi, H. et al. Hericenones C, D, and E, stimulators of Nerve Growth Factor synthesis, from the mushroom Hericium erinaceum. Tetrahedron Lett. 1991; 32, 4361-4564.
2. Kawagishi, H. et al. Chromans, Hericenones F, G, and H from the mushroom Hericium erinaceum. Phytochemistry. 1993; 32, 175-178.
3. Furukawa, S. et al. Biological Significance of Nerve Growth Factor and its Syntheses-Promoting Agent. Chemistry and Biology. 1991; 29. (In Japanese)
4. Kawagishi, H. The Basic Chemistry of Mushrooms and Fungus and Biotechnology, Shishido, K. (editor). 2002; IPC, 212-228. (In Japanese)
5. Kawagishi, H. Science of Mushrooms, Suguwara, R. (editor). Asakura Shoten. 1997; 155-180. (In Japanese)
6. Kawagishi, H. et al. Search for Bioregulating Agents of Edible Mushrooms and Their Performance Analysis, Arai, S. (editor). Gakkai Shuppann Center, 1995; 37-43.
7. Kawagishi, H. et al. The Inducer of the Synthesis of Nerve Growth Factor from Lion's Mane (Hericeum erinaceum). Explore! 2002; 11(4): 4-51.
8. Lee. E. W. et al. Two novel diterpenoids, erinacines H and I from the mycelia of Hericium erinaceum. Biosci. Biotechnol. Biochem. 2000; 64: 2402-2405
9. Kawagishi, H. et al. Erinacine D, a stimulator of NGF-synthesis, from the mycelia of Hericium erinaceum. Heterocycl. Commun. 1996; 2: 51-54.
10. Kawagishi, H. et al. Erinacines, E, F, and G, stimulators of nerve growth factor synthesis, from the mycelia of Hericium erinaceum. Tetrahedron Lett. 1996; 37: 7399-7402.
11. Kawagishi, H. et al Erinacines A, B, and C, strong stimulators of nerve growth factor synthesis, from the mycelia of Hericium erinaceum. Tetrahedron Lett. 1994; 35: 1569-1572
12. Kasahara, K. et al. The Benefits of Lion's Mane for Aged-disabled. Gunma Medical Supplementary issue. 2001; 77-81.
13. Granger, C. V., Hamilton, B. B., Linacre, J. M., Heinemann, A. W. and Wright, B. D.: Performance profiles of the functional independence measure, Am. J. Phys. Med. Rehabil. 72(2), 84-89 (1993).
14. Marino, R. J., Huang, M., Knight, P., Herbison, G. J., Ditunno, J. F. and Segal, M.: Assessing selfcare status in quardriplegia: comparison of the quadriplegia index of function (QIF) and the functional independence measure, Parsplegia 31, 225-233 (1993).

Maca

1. Vavilov, N. 1. The Origin, Variation, Immunity and Breeding of Cultivated Plants. (Waltham, Massachusetts: Smithsonian Institute, 1957) p. 364.
2. King, S.R. "Four endemic Andean tuber crops: Promising food resources for agricultural diversification." Mountain Research and Development. 7(l):432, 1987.
3. Chacon de Popvici, G. La importancia de Lepidium peruvianum Chacon (Maca) en

la Alimentacion y Salud del ser Humano y Animal 2,000 Anos Antes y Despues de Cristo y en el Siglo XXI. Peru, 1997.

4. Chacon, R.C., "Estudio fitoquimico de Lepidium meyenii Walp." Thesis Universidad Nacional. Mayor de San Marcos, Lima, Peru, 1961, p, 43.

5. Dini, A., et al, "Chemical Composition of Lepidium mayenii." Food Chemistry. 49:347-349, 1994.

6. Effect of Lepidium meyenii (Maca herb), a root with aphrodisiac and fertility-enhancing properties, on serum reproductive hormone levels in adult healthy men. J Endocrinol. 2003 Jan;176(1):163-8.

7. Effect of Lepidium meyenii (maca herb) on sexual desire and its absent relationship with serum testosterone levels in adult healthy men. Andrologia. 2002 Dec;34(6):367-72.

8. Smallanthus sonchifolius and Lepidium meyenii (maca herb) - prospective Andean crops for the prevention of chronic diseases. Biomed Pap Med Fac Univ Palacky Olomouc Czech Repub. 2003 Dec;147(2):119-30.

9. Lepidium meyenii (Maca root) improved semen parameters in adult men. Asian J Androl. 2001 Dec;3(4):301-3.

10. Red maca (Lepidium meyenii) reduced prostate size in rats. Reprod Biol Endocrinol. 2005 Jan 20;3(1):5.

11. Effect of Lepidium meyenii (Maca root) on spermatogenesis in male rats acutely exposed to high altitude. J Endocrinol. 2004 Jan;180(1):87-95.

12. Effect of alcoholic extract of Lepidium meyenii (Maca) on testicular function in male rats. Universidad Peruana Cayetano Heredia, Postal Office Lima, Peru.

13. Hexanic Maca extract improves rat sexual performance more effectively than methanolic and chloroformic Maca extracts. Andrologia. 2002 Jun;34(3):177-9.

14. Maca root improves sexual behavior in male rats independently from its action on spontaneous locomotor activity. J Ethnopharmacol. 2001 May;75(2-3):225-9.

15. Nutritional evaluation of Lepidium meyenii (Maca root) in albino mice and their descendants Arch Latinoam Nutr. 2000 Jun;50(2):126-33.

16. Imidazole alkaloids from Lepidium meyenii (maca extract). J Nat Prod. 2003 Aug;66(8):1101-3.

17. Canales M, Aguilar J, Prada A, Marcelo A, Huaman C, Carbajal L. Nutritional evaluation of Lepidium meyenii (MACA) in albino mice and their descendant. Arch Latinoam Nutr. 2000 Jun;50(2):126-33.

18. Chacon, G., 1990. La maca (Lepidium peruvianum) Chacon sp. Nov. Y su habitat. Revista Peruana de Biologia 3:171-272.

19. Dini, A., et.al., 199994., "Chemical composition of Lepidium meyenii," Food Chemistry 49: 347-349.

20. Gomez, A., "Maca, Es alternativa Nutricional para el ano 2000." Informe Ojo con su Salud No. 58 August 15, 1997, Lima Peru.

21. Johns, T. 1981. The anu and the maca. Journal of Ethnobiology, 1:208-212.

22. King, Steven, 1986. "Ancient Buried Treasure of the Andes," Garden, November/December.

23. Leon, J. 1964. The "maca" (Lepidium Meyenii) a little known food plant of Peru. Economic Botany. 18:122-127.

24. Quiros, C. et al., "Physiological Studies and Determination of Chromosome Number

in Maca, Lepidium Meyenii." Economic Botany 50(2) pp. 216-223. 1996.
25. Report of an Ad Hoc Panel of the Advisory Committee on Technical Innovation, Board on Science and Technology for International Development, National Research Council, 1989. Lost Crops of the Incas: Little Known Plants of the Andes with Promise for Worldwide Cultivation.

Maqui Berry

1. Experimental study of the effects of cyaninoside chloride on collagen, and its potential value in ophthalmology.
Miskulin M, Godeau G, Tixier AM, Robert AM.
J Fr Ophtalmol. 1984;7(11):737-43. French.
2. Effects of anthocyanins on psychological stress-induced oxidative stress and neurotransmitter status.
Rahman MM, Ichiyanagi T, Komiyama T, Sato S, Konishi T.
J Agric Food Chem. 2008 Aug 27;56(16):7545-50. Epub 2008 Jul 29.
3. Anthocyanins and heart health.
Mazza GJ.
Ann Ist Super Sanita. 2007;43(4):369-74. Review.
4. Evaluation and development of botanical drugs from Aristotelia Chilensis, Juan Hancke, Rafael Burgo. Universidad Chile Valdivia
5. Effects of Maqio berry (Aristotelia chilensis) on Inflammation.
Juan Hancke, Rafael Burgos. Universidad Chile Valdivia
6. Anthocyanins in berries of Maqui (Aristotelia chilensis (Mol.) Stuntz). Escribano-Bailón MT, Alcalde-Eon C, Muñoz O, Rivas-Gonzalo JC, Santos-Buelga C.
Published: Phytochem Anal. 2006 Jan-Feb;17(1):8-14.
7. Berry fruits: compositional elements, biochemical activities, and the impact of their intake on human health, performance, and disease. Seeram NP.
Published: J Agric Food Chem. 2008 Feb 13;56(3):627-9. Epub 2008 Jan 23.
8. Juice and phenolic fractions of the berry Aristotelia chilensis inhibit LDL oxidation in vitro and protect human endothelial cells against oxidative stress. Miranda-Rottmann S, Aspillaga AA, Pérez DD, Vasquez L, Martinez AL, Leighton F.
Published: J Agric Food Chem. 2002 Dec 18;50(26):7542-7.
9. Evaluation of the analgesic, anti-inflammatory, free radical scavenger and antimicrobial properties of Aristotelia chilensis leaves
Juan Hancke, Rafael Burgos. Universidad Chile Valdivia
10. Bioactives component in maqui and rose hip.
Juan Hancke, Rafael Burgo. Universidad Chile Valdivia
11. Bioavailability, antioxidant and biological properties of the natural free-radical scavengers cyanidin and related glycosides.
Galvano F, La Fauci L, Vitaglione P, Fogliano V, Vanella L, Felgines C.
Ann Ist Super Sanita. 2007;43(4):382-93.
12. Anthocyanins and anthocyanin-rich extracts: role in diabetes and eye function.
Ghosh D, Konishi T. Health and Food, The Horticulture and Food Research Institute of New Zealand Ltd., PB 92169, Auckland, New Zealand. Asia Pac J Clin Nutr. 2007;16(2):200-8.

13. Anthocyanins inhibit airway inflammation and hyperresponsiveness in a murine asthma model. Park SJ, Shin WH, Seo JW, Kim EJ.
Korea Institute of Toxicology, Korea Research Institute of Chemical Technology, Yuseong, Daejeon 305-600, Republic of Korea.
Food Chem Toxicol. 2007 Aug;45(8):1459-67. Epub 2007 Feb 20.

14. Anti-inflammatory effects of flavonoids in the natural juice from Aronia melanocarpa, rutin, and rutin-magnesium. Complex on an experimental model of inflammation induced by histamine and serotonin.
Borissova P, et al.
Acta Physiol Pharmacol Bulg 1994;20(1):25-30.

15. The relative antioxidant activities of plant-derived polyphenolic flavonoids.
Rice-Evans CA.
Free Radical Res 1995 Apr;22(4):3785-93.

16. Antioxidant activity of nasunin, an anthocyanin in eggplant peels.
Noda Y.
Toxicology 2000 Aug 7;148(2-3):119-23.

17. Inhibition of LDL oxidation by phenolic substances in red wine: a clue to the French paradox?
Nutr Rev. 1993 Jun;51(6):185-7.

18. Dietary flavanols and procyanidin oligomers from cocoa (Theobroma cacao) inhibit platelet function.
Murphy KJ, Chronopoulos AK, Singh I, Francis MA, Moriarty H, Pike MJ, Turner AH, Mann NJ, Sinclair AJ.
Am J Clin Nutr. 2003 Jun;77(6):1466-73.

19. Endothelin-1 synthesis reduced by red wine. Red wines confer extra benefit when it comes to preventing coronary heart disease.
William Harvey Research Institute, Barts & theLondon School of Medicine & Dentistry, Queen Nature, Vol 414, 20/27 December 2001

20. Activation of innate immunity system during aging: NF-kB signaling is the molecular culprit of inflamm-aging.
Salminen A, Huuskonen J, Ojala J, Kauppinen A, Kaarniranta K, Suuronen T.
Department of Neuroscience and Neurology, University of Kuopio, Kuopio, Finland. Ageing Res Rev. 2008 Apr;7(2):83-105. Epub 2007 Sep 20.

21. Cyclooxygenase-2 regulates mesenchymal cell differentiation into the osteoblast lineage and is critically involved in bone repair
Xinping Zhang1, Edward M. Schwarz1, Donald A. Young2, J. Edward Puzas1, Randy N. Rosier1 and Regis J. O'Keefe11 The Center for Musculoskeletal Research, University of Rochester Medical Center, and 2 Department of Medicine/ Endocrinology, University of Rochester School of Medicine and Dentistry, Rochester, New York, USA J. Clin. Invest. 109(11): 1405-1415 (2002).

22. Signalling networks regulating cyclooxygenase-2.
Tsatsanis C, Androulidaki A, Venihaki M, Margioris AN.
Int J Biochem Cell Biol. 2006;38(10):1654-61. Epub 2006 Apr 25. Review.

23. Comparison of Antioxidant Potency of Commonly Consumed Polyphenol-Rich Beverages in the United States
NAVINDRA P. SEERAM,† MICHAEL AVIRAM,§ YANJUN ZHANG,†

SUSANNE M. HENNING,† LYDIA FENG,† MARK DREHER,# AND DAVID HEBER*,†
J. Agric. Food Chem. 2008, 56, 1415–1422

Monolaurin

1. Fatty Acids and Derivatives as Antimicrobial Agents Antimicrobial Agents and Chemotherapy 2(l):23-28 (1972) Kabara. J.J.. Conley. A J.- Swieczkowski. D M. Ismail, I.A . Lie Ken Jie and Gunstone, F D Antimicrobial Action of Isomeric Fatty Acids on Group A Streptococcus Journal of Medicinal Chemistry 16:1060-1063 (1973).

2. Antimicrobial Lipids: Natural and Synthetic Fatty Acids and Monoglycerides. Kabara. J.J., Vrable, R. and Lie Ken Jie, M.S.F Lipids 12:753759 (1977).

3. Toxicological, Bactericidal and Fungicidal Properties of Fatty Acids and Some Derivatives Kabara, J.J. JAOCS 56:760-767

4. Lauric oils as antimicrobial agents: theory of effect, scientific rationale, and dietary applications as adjunct nutritional support for HIV-infected individuals in Nutrients and Foods in AIDS (RR Watson, ed) CRC Press, Boca Raton, 1998, pp. 81-97. Enig, MG

5. Glycerol monolaurate inhibits the effects of Gram-positive select agents on eukaryotic cells. Biochemistry. 2006 Feb 21;45(7):2387-97. Peterson ML, Schlievert PM

6. In vitro activity of lauric acid or myristylamine in combination with six antimicrobial agents against methicillin-resistant Staphylococcus aureus (MRSA). International Journal of Antimicrobrial Agents. 2006 Jan;27(1):51-7. Epub 2005 Nov 28. Kitahara T, Aoyama Y, Hirakata Y, Kamihira S, Kohno S, Ichikawa N, Nakashima M, Sasaki H, Higuchi S.

7. Glycerol monolaurate inhibits virulence factor production in Aacillus anthracis. Antimicrobial Agents and Chemotherapy. 2005 Apr;49(4):1302-5. Vetter SM, Schlievert PM.

8. Effect of glycerol monolaurate on bacterial growth and toxin production. Antimicrobial Agents Chemotherapy. 1992 Mar;36(3):626-31. Schlievert PM, Deringer JR, Kim MH, Projan SJ, Novick RP.

9. In vitro and in vivo evaluations of the activities of lauric acid monoester formulations against Staphylococcus aureus. Antimicrobial Agents Chemotherapy. 2005 Aug;49(8):3187-91. Rouse MS, Rotger M, Piper KE, Steckelberg JM, Scholz M, Andrews J, Patel R.

10. Antimicrobial activity of monocaprin: a monoglyceride with potential use as a denture disinfectant. Acta Odontol Scand. 2006 Feb;64(1):21-6. Thorgeirsdottir TO, Kristmundsdottir T, Thormar H, Axelsdottir I, Holbrook WP.

11. Development of a virucidal cream containing the monoglyceride monocaprin. Pharmazie. 2005 Dec;60(12):897-9. Thorgeirsdottir TO, Hilmarsson H, Thormar H, Kristmundsdottir T.

12. Stable concentrated emulsions of the 1-monoglyceride of capric acid (monocaprin) with microbicidal activities against the food-borne bacteria Campylobacter jejuni,

Salmonella spp., and Escherichia coli. Applied Environmental Microbiology. 2006 Jan;72(1):522-6. Thormar H, Hilmarsson H, Bergsson G.

13. Killing of Gram-positive cocci by fatty acids and monoglycerides. APMIS. 2001 Oct;109(10):670-8. Bergsson G, Arnfinnsson J, Steingrimsson O, Thormar H.

14. In vitro susceptibilities of Neisseria gonorrhoeae to fatty acids and monoglycerides. Antimicrobial Agents and Chemotherapy. 1999 Nov;43(11):2790-2. Bergsson G, Steingrimsson O, Thormar H.

15. In vitro inactivation of Chlamydia trachomatis by fatty acids and monoglycerides. Antimicrobial Agents and Chemotherapy. 1998 Sep;42(9):2290-4. Bergsson G, Arnfinnsson J, Karlsson SM, Steingrimsson O, Thormar H.

Probiotics

1. Kuwaki et al, Antifungal activity of the fermentation product of herbs by lactic acid bacteria against tinea, 2002, vol. 94 No. 5, pp. 401-405.*

2. Iichiro Ohhira et al., "Antimicrobial activity against methicillin-resistant Staphylococcus aureus in the culture broth of Enterococcus faecelis TH 10, an isolate from Malaysian fermentation food, Temph", Japanese Journal of Dairy and Food Science, vol. 45, No. 4, 1996.

3. Iichiro Ohhira et al., "Purification of Anti-Escherichia coli O-157 components produced by Enterococcus faecalis TH10, an isolate from Malaysian fermentation food, tempeh", Milk Science, vol. 49, No. 2, 2000.

4. Aim, L 1982. Effect of Fermentation on Lactose, Glucose and Galactose Content in Milk and Suitability of Fermented Milk Products for Lactose Intolerant Individuals. J. Dairy Sci., 65: 346-352

5. Gillilan). S. E., Nelson, C. R. & Maxwell. C. 1985. Assimilation ofCholesterol by Lactobacillus Acidophilus. Appl. Environ. Microbiol., 49: 377-381.

6. Gotz, V., Romankiemcz. J. A.. Moss, J. &Mwwy, H. W. 1979. Prophylaxis against Ampicillin-Associated Diairhea with a Lactobacillus Preparation. AmerJ. Hasp. Pharm., 36: 754.

7. Macbeth, W. A. A. G? Kass, E. H. &McDennolt. W. V. Jr. 1965. Treatment of Hepatic Encephalopathy by Alteration of Intestinal Flora with Lactobacillus acidophilus. Lancit., i: 399-403

8. Lilley, D. M. and StiUwell, R. H. (1965). Probiotics: growth promoting factors produced by Microorganisms. Science 147 747-748

9. Parker, R. B. (1974). Probiotics, the other half of the antibiotic story. Anim. Nutr. Health 29:4-8

10. Fuller, R. (1989). Probiotics in man and animals. J. Appl. Bacteriol. 66: 365-378

11. Hamdan, 1. Y. and Mikolajcik, E. M. (1974). Acidolin: an antibiotic produced by Lactobacillus acidophilus. Journal of Antibiotics 8: 631-636

12. R. Fuller, "Probiotics in Man and Animals," J. Appl. Bacteriol., 66: 365-378 (1989).

13. B.R. Goldin and S.L. Gorbach, "The Relationship Between Diet and Rat Faecal Enzymes Implicated in Colon Cancer," J. Natl. Cancer Inst., 57: 371-375 (1976).

14. B.R. Goldin and S.L. Gorbach, "Alterations in Faecal Microflora Enzymes Related to Diet, Age, Lactobacillus Supplements and Dimethylhydrazine," Cancer 40:2421-2426 (1977).
15. B.R. Goldin and S.L. Gorbach, "Alternations of the Intestinal Microflora by Diet, Oral Antibiotics and Lactobacillus: Decreased Production of Free Amines From Aromatic Nitro Compounds, Azo Dyes and Glucuronides," J. Natl. Cancer Inst., 73: 689-695 (1984a).
16. B.R. Goldin and S.L. Gorbach, "The Effect of Milk and Lactobacillus Feeding on Human Intestinal Bacterial Enzyme Activity." Amer. J. Clin. Nutr. 39: 756-761.
17. D.M. Lilley and R.H. Stillwell, "Probiotics: Growth Promoting Factors Produced by Microorganisms," Science 147: 747-748 (1965).
18. R.B. Parker, "Probiotics, the Other Half of the Antibiotic Story," Amin. Nutr. Health, 29: 4-8 (1974).
19. G.S. Sperti, "Probiotics," Avi Publishing Co., West Point, Connecticut (1971).

Resveratrol

1. Wine molecule slows aging process:Scientists drink to that. URL: http://www.news.harvard.edu/gazette/2003/09.18/12-antiaging.html [27 Dec 2004]
2. Pervaizi. Resveratrol: from grapevines to mammalian biology. The FASEB Journal. 2003;17:1975-1985
3. Natural Medicines Database Resveratrol Monograph URL: http://www.therapeuticresearch.net/(1wuptiicjogau4bo3n5yrb55)/nd/Search.aspx?rn=4&li=1&st=1&cs=&s=ND&pt=100&sh=4&id=307 [29 Dec 2004]
4. Natural Medicines Database Wine Monograph URL: http://www.therapeuticresearch.net/(1wuptiicjogau4bo3n5yrb55)/nd/Search.aspx?rn=4&li=1&st=1&cs=&s=ND&pt=100&sh=2&id=989 [29 Dec 2004]
5. Xiao K et al. Constituents from Polygonum cuspidatum. Chem Pharm Bull 2002 May;50(5):605-8
   Japanese Knotweed (Polygonum cuspidatum). URL: http://ipcm.wisc.edu/uw_weeds/extension/articles/japknotweed.htm [Dec 27 2004]
6. Lamming et al. Small molecules that regulate lifespan: evidence for xenohormesis. Molecular Microbiology 2004 53(4) 1003-1009
7. Howitz et al. Small molecule activators of sirtuins extend Saccharomyces cerevisiae lifespan. Nature. September 2003 425:191-196
8. Jennifer Couzin. Aging Research's Family Feud. Science Feb 2004 303:1276-1279
9. Wood et al. Sirtuin activators mimic caloric restriction and delay ageing in metazoans. Nature September 2004 430(7000):686-9
10. Stivala L et al. Specific Structural Determinants Are Responsible for the Antioxidant Activity and the Cell Cycle Effects of Resveratrol. J of Biological Chemistry 2001 276(25):22586-22594
11. Noroozi et al. Effects of flavonoids and vitamin C on oxidative DNA damage to human lymphocytes. Am J Clin Nutr. 1998 67:1210-8
12. Anderson et al. Nicotinamide and PNC1 govern lifespan extension by calorie restriction in Saccharomyces cerevisiae. Nature May 2003 423:181-185 2

13. An Open Letter To Consumers and manufacturers of Resveratrol Dietary Supplements, from Longevinex™. URL: http://www.longevinex.com/sdm.asp?pg=ol [29 Dec 2004]

14. Kodan A et al. A stibene synthase from Japanese red pine (Pinus densiflora): Implications for phytoalexin accumlation and down-regulation of flavonoid biosynthesis. PNAS 2002 99(5) 3335-3339

15. Chiron H et al. Gene Induction of Stilbene Biosynthesis in Scots Pine in Response to Ozone Treatment, Wounding, and Fungal Infection. Plant Physiology 2000 124:865-872

16. Guarente, Leonard. Sir2 links chromatin silencing, metabolism, and aging. Genes & Development 2000 14:1021-1026

17. De Santi C et al. Sulphation of resveratrol, a natural compound found in wine, and its inhibition by natural flavonoids. Xenobiotica 2000 Sep 30(9) 857-66

18. De Santi C et al. Glucuronidation of resveratrol, a natural product present in grape and wine, in human liver. Xenobiotica 2000 Nov 30(11) 1047-54

19. Marier J-F et al. Metabolism and Disposition of Resveratrol in Rats: Extent of Absorption, Glucuronidation, and Enteroheptic Recirculation Evidenced by a Linked-Rat Model The Journal of Pharmacology and Experimental Therapeutics. 2002 302:369-373

20. Andreas J. et al. Relationship between Mechanisms, Bioavailibility, and Preclinical Chemopreventive Efficacy of Resveratrol: A Conundrum Cancer Epidemiology Biomarkers & Prevention Vol. 12, 953-957, October 2003

21. Raucy J. Regulation of CYP3A4 Expression in Human Hepatocytes by Pharmaceuticals and Natural Products. Drug Metabolism and Disposition. 2003 31(5) 533-539

22. Juan ME et al.The Daily Oral Administration of High Doses of trans-Resveratrol to Rats for 28 Days Is Not Harmful. American Society for Nutritional Sciences. 2002 132:257-260

23. FDA Letter of New Dietary Ingredient Resveratrol. URL: http://www.fda.gov/ohrms/dockets/dockets/95s0316/rpt0085_01.pdf [07 JAN 2005]

24. FDA Letter of New Dietary Ingredient trans-Resveratrol. URL: http://www.fda.gov/ohrms/dockets/dockets/95s0316/95s-0316-rpt0101-web.pdf [07 JAN 2005] 3

25. Farley. (2003). Cytotoxic pharmaceutical composition. US Patent 6,544,564

26. Toppo. (2000). Treatment for blood cholesterol with trans-resveratrol. US Patent 6,048,903

27. Farley (2004). Immune functions. US Patent 6,767,563

28. Pharmascience Inc (2001). Administration of resveratrol to prevent or treat restenosis following coronary intervention. US Patent 6,022,901

29. Pharmascience Inc (1998). Cancer chemopreventative composition and method. US Patent 6,008,260

30. Cavazza (1998). Pharmaceutical composition comprising L-carnitine or derivative thereof and trihydroxy or tetrahydroxystilbene. US Patent 5,747,536

31. Hao et al. Mechanism of cardiovascular protection by resveratrol. J Med Food. 2004 7(3):290-8

32. Wang Z et al. Effect of resveratrol on platelet aggregation in vivo and in vitro. Chin Med J. 2002 115(3):378-80

33. Pace Asciak et atl. The red wine phenolics trans-resveratrol and quercetin block human platelet aggreagation and eicosanoid synthesis: implicatiosn for protection against coronary heart disease. Clin Chim Acta 1995 235(2):207-19

34. Turner et al. Is resveratrol an estrogen agonist in growing rats? Endocrinology 1999 140(1):50-4

35. Jiangang et al. Effects of resveratrol on oxidative modification on human low density lipoprotein Chin Med J 2000;113(2):99-102

36. Estrov Z et al. Resveratrol blocks interleukin-1B-induced activation of the nuclear transcription factor NF-kB, inhibits proliferation, causes S-phase arrest, and induced apoptosis of acute myeloid leukemia cells. Blood. 2003 102:987-995

37. Manna et al. Resveratrol suppresses TNF-Induced Activation of Nuclear Transcription Factors NF-kB, Activator Protein-1, and Apoptosis: Potential Role of Reactive Oxygen Intermediates and Lipid Peroxidation. J. of Immunology 2000 164:6509-6519

38. Pellegatta et al. Different short- and long-term effects of resveratrol on nuclear factor-kB phosphorylation and nuclear appearance in human endothelial cells. Am J Clin Nutr 2003 77:1220-8 4

39. McElwee et al. Shared Transcriptional Signature in Caenorhabditis elegans Dauer Larvae and Long-lived daf-2 Mutants Implicates Detoxification System in Longevity Assurance. J Biological Chemistry. 2004 43:44533-44543

40. Nigdikar et al. Consumption of red wine polyphenols reduces the susceptibility of low-density lipoproteins to oxidation in vivo. Am J Clin Nutr. 1998 68:258-65

41. Leung, A.Y. (1996). Encyclopedia of Common Natural Ingredients Used in Food, Drugs, And Cosmetics Second Edition. New York, John Wiley & Sons

42. Natural Medicines Database Green Tea Monograph URL: http://www. therapeuticresearch.net/(1wuptiicjogau4bo3n5yrb55)/nd/Search.aspx? li=1&st=2& cs=&s=ND&pt=100&sh=0&id=960 [20 June 2005]

43. Kaeberlein et al. Substrate-specific activation of sirtuins by resveratrol. J Biol Chem 2005. 280:17038-45

44. Srinivas, Babykutty, Sathiadevan, Srinivas. Molecular mechanism of emodin action: Transition from laxative ingredient to an antitumor agent. Med Res Rev. 2006. [Epub ahead of print]

45. Jahnke, Price, Marr, Myers, George. Developmental toxicity evaluation of emodin in rats and mice. Birth Defects Res B Dev Reprod Toxicol. 2004. 71(2): 89-101

46. Kaneshiro, Morioka, Inamine, Kinjo, Arakaki, Chiba, Sunagawa, Suzui, Yoshimi. Anthroquinone derivative emodin inhibits tumor-associated angiogenesis through inhibitionof extracellular signal regulated kinase ½ phosphorylation. Eur J Pharmacol. 2006. 553(1-3):46-53

47. Olsen, Bjorling-Poulsen, Guerra. Emodin negatively affects the phosphoinositide 3-kinase/AKT signaling pathway: A study on its mechanism of action. Int J Biochem Cell Biol. 2007. 39(1): 227-37

48. Garg, Buchholz, Aggarwal. Chemosensitization and radiosensitization of tumors by plant polyphenols. Antioxid Redox Signal. 2005 7(11-12): 1630-47

49. US Dept. of Health and Human Services, NIH, National Toxicology Program Technical Report. NTP Toxicology and Carcinogenesis Studies of EMODIN (CAS NO. 518-82-1) Feed Studies in F344/N Rats and B6C3F1 Mice. 2001 493:1-278. http://ntp.niehs.nih.gov/ntp/htdocs/LT_rpts/tr493.pdf accessed 12/28/2006.

50. Jang M, Cai L, Udeani GO, et al. Cancer chemopreventive activity of resveratrol, a natural product derived from grapes. Science 1997;275:218-20. 5

51. Hascalik S, Celik O, Turkoz Y, et al. Resveratrol, a red wine constituent polyphenol, protects from ischemia-reperfusion damage of the ovaries. Gynecol Obstet Invest 2004;57:218-23.

52. Soleas GJ, Diamandis EP, Goldberg DM. Resveratrol: a molecule whose time has come? And gone? Clin Biochem 1997;30:91-113.

53. Bertelli AA, Giovannini L, Bernini W, et al. Antiplatelet activity of cisresveratrol. Drugs Exp Clin Res 1996;22:61-3.

54. Pace-Asciak CR, Rounova O, Hahn SE, et al. Wines and grape juices as modulators of platelet aggregation in healthy human subjects. Clin Chim Acta 1996;246:163-82.

55. Bertelli A, et al. Plasma and tissue resveratrol concentrations and pharmacological activity. Drugs Exp Clin Res, 1998; 24(3): 133-8.

56. Bertelli AA, et al. Antiplatelet activity of synthetic and natural resveratrol in red wine. Int J Tissue React 1995;17:1-3.

57. Personal correspondence between Stephen Sturm, Senior Project Manager and Dr. Sato of the Institution of Enology and Viticulture, University of Yamanashi 13-1, Kitashin 1-chome, Kofu 400-0005 JAPAN phone: +81-55-220-8769 fax; +81-55-220-8768 E-mail: msatoh@yamanashi.ac.jp.

58. CHEMICALS KNOWN TO THE STATE TO CAUSE CANCER OR REPRODUCTIVE TOXICITY DECEMBER 8, 2006 http://www.oehha.ca.gov/prop65/prop65_list/files/P65single120806.pdf

59. Valenzano DR,, et. al. Resveratrol prolongs lifespan and retards the onset of age-related markers in a short-lived vertebrate. Curr Biol. 2006 Feb 7;16(3):296-300.

60. Baur JA, et. al. Resveratrol improves health and survival of mice on a high-calorie diet. Nature. 2006 Nov 16;444(7117):337-42. Epub 2006 Nov 1.

61. Resveratrol Prolongs Lifespan And Delays The Onset Of Aging-related Traits In A Short-lived Vertebrate. Medical News Today. http://www.medicalnewstoday.com/medicalnews.php?newsid=38094 [17 JAN 2007]

62. FDA Cyber Warning Letter to Douglas Labs. http://www.fda.gov/cder/warn/cyber/2002/CFSANdouglaslabs.htm [17 JAN 2007] 6

63. Red wine compound may extend life, says mice study. Nutra Ingredients Europe. http://www.nutraingredients.com/news/ng.asp?n=71767-resveratrol-red-winesurvival.
[2 NOV 2006]

64. FDA Cyber Warning Letter to VP Nutrition. http://www.fda.gov/cder/warn/cyber/2005/CL168e.pdf [18 JAN 2007]

65. FDA Warning Letter to Ocean Spray Cranberries, Inc. http://www.fda.gov/foi/warning_letters/m5075n.pdf [18 JAN 2007]

66. USDA Agricultural Research Service Phytochemical Database http://www.arsgrin. gov/duke/ [18 JAN 2007]
67. Natural Medicines Database Senna Monograph URL: http://www.naturaldatabase. com/(S(0nqh44453dgujp55rdhznt55))/nd/Search.aspx ?cs=&s=ND&pt=100&id=652&fs=ND&searchid=3029587 [18 JAN 2007]
68. McGuffin M, Hobbs C, Upton R, Goldberg A, eds. American Herbal Products Association's Botanical Safety Handbook. Boca Raton, FL: CRC Press, LLC 1997.
69. Emodin ChemExper Chemical Directory. http://www.chemexper.com/chemicals/ supplier/cas/518-82-1.html [2 FEB 2007]
70. Warning Letter to Pavich Family Farms. http://www.fda.gov/foi/warning_letters/ m5016n.pdf

Ribose

1. Andreoli S. Mechanisms of endothelial cell ATP depletion after oxidant injury. Pediatric Res 1989;25(1):97-100.
2. Angello D, R Wilson, D Gee, N Perlmutter. Recovery of myocardial function and thallium 201 redistribution using ribose. Am J Card Imag 1989;3(4):256-265.
3. Asimakis G, J Zwischenberger, K Inners-McBride, L Sordahl, V Conti. Postischemic recovery of mitochondrial adenine nucleotides in the heart. Circ 1992;85(6):2212-2220.
4. Baldwin D, E McFalls, D Jaimes, P Fashingbauer, T Nemzek, H Ward. Myocardial glucose metabolism and ATP levels are decreased two days after global ischemia. J Surg Res 1996;63:35-38.
5. Befera N, A Rivard, D Gatlin, S Black, J Zhang, JE Foker. Ribose treatment helps preserve function of the remote myocardium after myocardial infarction. J Surg Res 2007;137(2):156.
6. Brault JJ, RL Terjung. Purine salvage to adenine nucleotides in different skeletal muscle fiber types. J Appl Physiol 2001;91:231-238.
7. Carter O, D MacCarter, S Mannebach, J Biskupiak, G Stoddard, EM Gilbert, MA Munger. D-Ribose improves peak exercise capacity and ventilatory efficiency in heart failure patients. JACC 2005;45(3 Suppl A):185A.
8. Chatham J, R Challiss, G Radda, A Seymour. Studies of the protective effect of ribose in myocardial ischaemia by using 31P-nuclear magnetic resonance spectroscopy. Biochem Soc Proc 1985;13:885-888.
9. Clay MA, P Stewart-Richardson, D Tasset, J Williams. Chronic alcoholic cardiomyopathy: Protection of the isolated ischemic working heart by ribose. Biochem Internat 1988;17(5):791-800.
10. Cohen M, R Charney, R Hershman, V Fuster, R Gorlin, X Francis. Reversal of chronic ischemic myocardial dysfunction after transluminal coronary angioplasty. JACC 1988;12(5):1193-1198.
11. Dodd SL, CA Johnson, K Fernholz, JA St.Cyr. The role of ribose in human skeletal muscle metabolism. Med Hypoth 2004;62(5):819-824.
12. Dow J, S Nigdikar, J Bowditch. Adenine nucleotide synthesis de novo in mature rat cardiac myocytes. Biochim Biophys Acta 1985;847(2):223-227.

13. Einzig S, JA St.Cyr, R Bianco, J Schneider, E Lorenz, J Foker. Myocardial ATP repletion with ribose infusion. Pediatr Res 1985;19:127A.

14. Einzig S, J St. Cyr, J Schneider, R Bianco, J Foker. Maintained myocardial ATP with long term ribose. Pediatr Res 1986;20(4 pt 2):169A.

15. Gao W, Y Liu, E Marban. Selective effects of oxygen free radicals on excitation-contraction coupling in ventricular muscle. Circ 1996;94: 2597-2604.

16. Gebhart B, J Jorgenson. Benefit of ribose in a patient with fibromyalgia. Pharm 2004;24(11):1646-1648.

17. Geisbuhler T, T Schwager. Ribose-enhanced synthesis of UTP, CTP, and GTP from parent nucleosides in cardiac myocytes. J Mol Cell Cardiol 1998;30(4):879-887.

18. Goncalves RP, GC Bennet, CP Leblond. Fate of 3H-ribose in the rat as detected by autoradiography. Anat Rec 1969;165:543-557.

19. Gradus-Pizlo I, SG Sawada, S Lewis, S Khouri, DS Segar, R Kovacs, H Feigenbaum. Effect of D-ribose on the detection of the hibernating myocardium during the low dose dobutamine stress echocardiography. Circ 1999;100(18):3394.

20. Grant GF, RW Gracey. Therapeutic nutraceutical treatments for osteoarthritis and ischemia. Exp Opin Ther Patents 2000;10(1): 1-10.

21. Griffiths JC, JF Borzelleca, J St. Cyr. Sub-chronic (13-week) oral toxicity study with D-ribose in Wistar rats. Food Chem Toxicol 2007;45(1):1440152.

22. Griffiths JC, JF Borzelleca, J St. Cyr. Lack of oral embryotoxicity/teratogenicity with D-ribose in Wistar rats. Food Chem Toxicol 2007; 45(3):388-395.

23. Gross G, J Auchampac. Role of ATP dependent potassium channels in myocardial ischaemia. Cardiovasc Res 1992;26:1011-1016.

24. Gross M, S Reiter, N Zollner. Metabolism of D-ribose administered to healthy persons and to patients with myoadenylate deaminase deficiency. Klin Wochenschr 1989;67:1205-1213.

25. Gross M, B Dormann, N Zollner. Ribose administration during exercise: effects on substrates and products of energy metabolism in healthy subjects and a patient with myoadenylate deaminase deficiency. Klin Wochenschr 1991;69:151-155.

26. Haas G, L DeBoer, E O'Keefe, R Bodenhamer, G Geffin, L Drop, R Teplick, W Daggett. Reduction of postischemic myocardial dysfunction by substrate repletion during reperfusion. Circ 1984;70:165-174.

27. Harmsen E, PP de Tombe, JW de Jong, PW Achterberg. Enhanced ATP and GTP synthesis from hypoxanthine or inosine after myocardial ischemia. Am J Physiol 1984;246 (1 Pt 2):H37-43.

28. Hegewald MG, RT Palac, D Angello, NS Perlmutter, RA Wilson. Ribose infusion accelerates thallium redistribution with early imaging compared with late 24-hour imaging without ribose. J Am Coll Cardiol 1991;18:1671-1681.

29. Hellsten Y, L Skadgauge, J Bangsbo. Effect of ribose supplementation on resynthesis of adenine nucleotides after intense intermittent training in humans. Am J Physiol 2004;286(1):R182-R188.

30. Ibel H, HG Zimmer. Metabolic recovery following temporary regional myocardial ischemia in the rat. J Mol Cell Cardiol 1986;18(Suppl 4):61-65.

31. Illien S, H Omran, D MacCarter, J St. Cyr. Ribose improves myocardial function in congestive heart failure. FASEB J 2001;15(5):A1142.

32. Ingwall JS. ATP and the Heart. Kluwer Academic Publishers, Boston, Massachusetts. 2002.

33. Ingwall JS, RG Weiss. Is the failing heart energy starved? On using chemical energy to support cardiac function. Circ Res 2004;95(2):135-45.

34. Kalsi K, R Smolenski, M Yacoub. Effects of nucleoside transport inhibitors and adenine/ribose supply on ATP concentration and adenosine production in cardiac myocytes. Moll Cell Biochem 1998;180(1-2):193-199.

35. Karnicki K, C Johnson, J St. Cyr, D Ericson, G Rao. Platelet storage solution improves the in vitro function of preserved platelet concentrate. Vox Sang 2003;85: 262-268.

36. Keith M. Increased oxidative stress in patients with congestive heart failure. J Am Coll Cardiol 1998;31(6):1352-1356.

37. Koumi S, R Martin, R Sato. Alterations in ATP-sensitive potassium channel sensitivity to ATP in failing human hearts. Am J Physiol 1997;272(41):H1656-H1665.

38. Lanoue K, J Watts, C Koch. Adenine nucleotide transport during cardiac ischemia. Am J Physiol 1981;24:H663-H671.

39. Lewandowski E, X Yu, K LaNoue, L White, C Doumen, M O'Donnell. Altered metabolic exchange between subcellular compartments in intact postischemic rabbit hearts. Circ Res 1997;81:165-175.

40. Lortet S, HG Zimmer. Functional and metabolic effects of ribose in combination with prazosin, verapamil and metroprolol in rats in vivo. Cardiovasc Res 1989;23:702-708.

41. Mahoney J, E Sako, K Seymour, C Marquardt, J Foker. A comparison of different carbohydrates as substrates for the isolated working heart. J Surg Res 1989;47:530-534.

42. Mahoney J. Recovery of postischemic myocardial ATP levels and hexosemonophosphate shunt activity. Med Hypoth 1990;31:21-23.

43. Mauser M, H Hoffmeister, C Nienaber, W Schaper. Influence of ribose, adenosine and "AICAR" on the rate of myocardial adenosine triphosphate synthesis during reperfusion after coronary artery occlusion in the dog. Circ Res 1985;56:220-230.

44. McDonagh TA, C Morrison, A Lawrence. Symptomatic and asymptomatic left-ventricular systolic dysfunction in an urban population. Lancet 1997;35:829-833.

45. Muller C, H Zimmer, M Gross, U Gresser, I Brotsack, M Wehling, W Pliml. Effect of ribose on cardiac adenine nucleotides in a donor model for heart transplantation. Eur J Med Res 1998;3:554-558.

46. Omran H, S Illien, D MacCarter, JA St. Cyr. Ribose improves myocardial function and quality of life in congestive heart failure patients. J Mol Cell Cardiol 2001;33(6):A173.

47. Omran H, S Illien, D MacCarter, JA St. Cyr, B Luderitz. D-Ribose improves diastolic function and quality of life in congestive heart failure patients: A prospective feasibility study. Eur J Heart Failure 2003;5:615-619.

48. Omran H, D MacCarter, JA St. Cyr, B Luderitz. D-Ribose aids congestive heart failure patients. Exp Clin Cardiol 2004;9(2):117-118.

49. Pasque M, T Spray, G Peliom, P van Trigt, R Peyton, W Currie, A Wechsler.

Ribose-enhanced myocardial recovery following ischemia in the isolated working rat heart. J Thorac Cardiovasc Surg 1982;83(3):390-398.

50. Pasque M, A Wechsler. Metabolic intervention to affect myocardial recovery following ischemia. Ann Surg 1984;200:1-10.

51. Patton BM. Beneficial effect of D-ribose in patient with myoadenylate deaminase deficiency. Lancet 1982 May8;1(8280):1701.

52. Pauly D, C Pepine. D-Ribose as a supplement for cardiac energy metabolism. J Cardiovasc Pharmacol Ther 2000;5(4):249-258.

53. Pauly D, C Johnson, JA St. Cyr. The benefits of ribose in cardiovascular disease. Med Hypoth 2003;60(2):149-151.

54. Pauly DF, CJ Pepine. Ischemic heart disease: Metabolic approaches to management. Clin Cardiol 2004;27(8):439-441.

55. Perkowski D, S Wagner, A Marcus, J St. Cyr. Pre-surgical loading of oral d-ribose improves cardiac index in patients undergoing "off pump" coronary artery revascularization. FASEB J 2005;19(4)Part1:A695.

56. Perkowski D, S Wagner, A Marcus, J St. Cyr. D-Ribose improves cardiac indicies in patients undergoing "off" pump coronary arterial revascularization. J Surg Res 2007;137(2):295.

57. Perkowski D, S Wagner, A Marcus, J St. Cyr. Ribose enhances ventricular function following off pump coronary artery bypass surgery. J Alt Comp Med 2005;11(4):745

58. Perlmutter NS, RA Wilson, DA Angello, RT Palac, J Lin, BG Brown. Ribose facilitates thallium-201 redistribution in patients with coronary artery disease. J Nucl Med 1991;32:193-200.

59. Pliml W, T von Arnim, A Stablein, H Hofmann, HG Zimmer, E Erdmann. Effects of ribose on exercise-induced ischaemia in stable coronary artery disease. Lancet 1992;340:507-510.

60. Pliml W, T von Arnim, C Hammer. Effects of therapeutic ribose levels on human lymphocyte proliferation in vitro. Clin Investig 1993;71(10):770-773.

61. Pouleur H. Diastolic dysfunction and myocardial energetics. Eur Heart J 1990;11(Supp C):30-34.

62. Redfield MM, SJ Jacobson, JC Burnett, DW Mahoney, KR Bailey, RJ Rodenheffer. Burden of systolic and diastolic ventricular dysfunction in the community. Appreciating the scope of the heart failure epidemic. JAMA 2003;289(2):194-202.

63. Reibel D, M Rovetto. Myocardial ATP synthesis and mechanical function following oxygen deficiency. Am J Physiol 1978;234(5):H620-H624.

64. Reimer K, M Hill, R Jennings. Prolonged depletion of ATP and of the adenine nucleotide pool due to delayed resynthesis of adenine nucleotides following reversible myocardial ischemic injury in dogs. J Mol Cell Cardiol 1981;13:229-239.

65. Salerno C, M Celli, R Finocchiaro, P D'Eufemia, P Iannetti, C Crifo, O Giardini. Effect of D-Ribose Administration to a patient with inherited deficit of Adenylosuccinase. Adv Exp Med Biol 1998;431:177-180.

66. Salerno C, P D'Eufemia, R Finocchiaro, M Celli, A Spalice, C Crifo, O Giardini. Effect of D-ribose on purine synthesis and neurological symptoms in a patient with

adenylsuccinase deficiency. Biochim Biophys Acta 1999;1453:135-140.

67. Sami H, N Bittar. The effect of ribose administration on contractile recovery following brief periods of ischemia. Anesthesiol 1987;67(3A):A74.

68. Schneider J, J St. Cyr, J Mahoney, R Bianco, W Ring, J Foker. Recovery of ATP and return of function after global ischemia. Circ 1985;72(4 pt 2):III-298.

69. Segal S, J Foley. The metabolism of D-ribose in man. J Clin Invest 1958;37:719-735.

70. Seifert J, A Subudhi, M-X Fu, K Riska, J John. The effects of ribose ingestion on indices of free radical production during hypoxic exercise. Free Rad Biol Med 2002;33(suppl 1):S269.

71. Sharma R, M Munger, S Litwin, O Vardeny, D MacCarter, JA St. Cyr. D-Ribose improves Doppler TEI myocardial performance index and maximal exercise capacity in stage C heart failure. J Mol Cell Cardiol 2005;38(5):853.

72. Siess M, U Delabar, H Seifart. Cardiac synthesis and degradation of pyridine nucleotides and the level of energy-rich phosphates influenced by various precursors. Adv Myocardiol 1983;4:287-308.

73. Skadhauge-Jensen L, J Bangsbo, Y Hellsten. Availability of ribose is limiting for ATP resynthesis in human skeletal after high-intensity training. Med Sci Sport Exc 2001;33(5).

74. Smolenski R, K Kalsi, M Zych, Z Kochan, M Yacoub. Adenine/ribose supply increases adenosine production and protects ATP pool in adenosine kinase-inhibited cardiac cells. J Mol Cell Cardiol 1998;30(3):673-683.

75. Smolenski R, K Kalsi, M Zych, Z Kochan, M Yacoub. Effects of adenine/ribose supply on adenosine production and ATP concentration in adenosine kinase-inhibited cardiac cells. Adv Exp Med Biol 1998;431:385-388.

76. Smolenski R, J Jayakumar, AM Seymour, MH Yacoub. High-energy phosphate changes in the normal and hypertrophied heart during cardioplegic arrest and ischemia. Adv Exp Med Biol 1998;431:286-286.

77. St. Cyr J, R Bianco, J Foker. Myocardial high-energy phosphate levels in cardiomyopathic turkeys. J Surg Res 1986;41:256-259.

78. St. Cyr J, H Ward, J Kriett, D Alyono, S Einzig, R Bianco, R Anderson, J Foker. Long-term model for evaluation of myocardial metabolic recovery following global ischemia. Adv Exp Med Biol 1986;194:401-441.

79. St. Cyr J, R Bianco, J Schneider, J Mahoney, K Tveter, S Einzig, J Foker. Enhanced high energy phosphate recovery with ribose infusion after global myocardial ischemia in a canine model. J Surg Res 1989;46(2):157-162.

80. Swain JL, R Sabina, P McHale, J Greenfield, E Holmes. Prolonged myocardial nucleotide depletion after brief ischemia in the open-chest dog. Am J Physiol 1982;242:H818-H826.

81. Taegtmeyer H, A Roberts, A Raine. Energy metabolism in reperfused heart muscle: Metabolic correlates to return of function. JACC 1985;6(4):864-870.

82. Taegtmeyer H, L King, B Jones. Energy substrate metabolism, myocardial ischemia and targets for pharmacotherapy. Am J Cardiol 1998;82(5A):54K-60K.

83. Taegtmeyer H. Metabolism - The lost child of cardiology. J Am Coll Cardiol 2000;36(4):1386-1388.

84. Tan ZT. Ruthenium red, ribose and adenine enhance recovery of reperfused rat heart. Coronary Artery Dis 1993;4(3):305-309.

85. Teitelbaum JE, C Johnson, J St Cyr. The use of D-ribose in chronic fatigue syndrome and fibromyalgia: a pilot study. J Altern Complement Med. 2006;12(9):857-62.

86. Tullson PC, RL Terjung. Adenine nucleotide synthesis in exercising and endurance-trained skeletal muscle. Am J Physiol 1991;261:C342-C347.

87. Tveter K, J St. Cyr, J Schneider, R Bianco, J Foker. Enhanced recovery of diastolic function after global myocardial ischemia in the intact animal. Pediatr Res 1988;23:226A.

88. Vance R, S Einzig, K Kreisler, J St. Cyr. D-Ribose maintains ejection fraction following aortic valve surgery. FASEB J 2000;14(4):A419.

89. Van Gammeren D, D Faulk, J Antonio. The effects of four weeks of ribose supplementation on body composition and exercise performance in healthy, young male recreational bodybuilders: A double-blind, placebo-controlled trial. Curr Ther Res 2002;63(8):486-495.

90. Vijay N, D MacCarter, M Washam, J St.Cyr. Ventilatory efficiency improves with d-ribose in congestive Heart Failure patients. J Mol Cell Cardiol 2005;38(5):820.

91. Wagner DR, U Gresser, N Zollner. Effects of oral ribose on muscle metabolism during bicycle ergometer in AMPD-deficient patients. Ann Nutr Metab 1991;35:297-302.

92. Wallen JW, MP Belanger, C Wittnich. Preischemic administration of ribose to delay the onset of irreversible ischemic injury and improve function: studies in normal and hypertrophied hearts. Can J Physiol Pharmacol 2003;81:40-47.

93. Ward H, J St. Cyr, J Cogordan, D Alyono, R Bianco, J Kriett, J Foker. Recovery of adenine nucleotide levels after global myocardial ischemia in dogs. Surgery 1984;96(2):248-255.

94. Williamson DL, PM Gallagher, MP Goddard, SW Trappe. Effects of ribose supplementation on adenine nucleotide concentration in skeletal muscle following high-intensity exercise. Med Sci Sport Exc 2001;33(5 suppl).

95. Wilson R, D MacCarter, J St. Cyr. D-Ribose enhances the identification of hibernating myocardium. Heart Drug 2003:3:61-62.

96. Wyatt D, S Ely, R Lasley, R Walsh, R Mainwaring, R Berne, R Mentzer. Purine-enriched asanguineous cardioplegia retards adenosine triphosphate degradation during ischemia and improves postischemic ventricular function. J Thorac Cardiovsac Res 1989;97:771-778.

97. Zarzeczny R, JJ Brault, KA Abraham, CR Hancock, RL Terjung. Influence of ribose on adenine salvage after intense muscle contractions. J Appl Physiol 2001;91:1775-1781.

98. Zimmer HG, E Gerlach. Stimulation of myocardial adenine nucleotide biosynthesis by pentoses and pentitols. Pflugers Arch 1978;376:223-227.

99. Zimmer HG. Restitution of myocardial adenine nucleotides: Acceleration by administration of ribose. J Physiol (Paris) 1980;76:769-775.

100. Zimmer HG, H Ibel, G Steinkopff. Studies on the hexose monophosphate shunt in the myocardium during development of hypertrophy. Adv Myocardiol 1980;1:487-

492.

101. Zimmer H-G, H Ibel, G Steinkopff, G Korb. Reduction of the isoproterenol-induced alterations in cardiac adenine nucleotides and morphology by ribose. Science 1980;207:319-321.

102. Zimmer HG. Normalization of depressed heart function in rats by ribose. Science 1983;220:81-82.

103. Zimmer HG, H Ibel. Effects of ribose on cardiac metabolism and function in isoproterenol-treated rats. Am J Physiol 1983;245:H880-H886.

104. Zimmer HG, H Ibel. Ribose accelerates the repletion of the ATP pool during recovery from reversible ischemia of the rat myocardium. J Mol Cell Cardiol 1984;16:863-866.

105. Zimmer HG, H Ibel, G Steinkopff. Ribose prevents the propranolol-induced reduction of myocardial adenine nucleotide biosynthesis. Adv Exp Med Biol 1984;165(Pt B):477-481.

106. Zimmer HG, H Ibel, U Suchner. Ribose intervention in the cardiac pentose phosphate pathway is not species-specific. Science 1984;223:712-714.

107. Zimmer HG, W Zierhut, G Marschner. Combination of ribose with calcium antagonist and beta-blocker treatment in closed-chest rats. J Mol Cell Cardiol 1987;19:635-639.

108. Zimmer HG, PA Martius, G Marschner. Myocardial infarction in rats: Effects of metabolic and pharmacologic interventions. Basic Res Cardiol 1989;84:332-343.

109. Zimmer HG. The oxidative pentose phosphate pathway in the heart: regulation, physiological significance and clinical implications. Basic Res Cardiol. 1992; 87: 3003-316.

110. Zimmer HG. Regulation of and intervention into the oxidative pentose phosphate pathway and adenine nucleotide metabolism in the heart. Mol Cell Biochem 1996;160-161:101-109.

111. Zimmer HG. Significance of the 5-phosphoribosyl-1-pyrophosphate pool for cardiac purine and pyrimidine nucleotide synthesis: studies with ribose, adenine, inosine, and orotic acid in rats. Cardiovasc Drug Ther 1998;12(Suppl 2):179-187.

112. Zollner N, S Reiter, M Gross, D Pongratz, CD Reimers, K Gerbitz, I Paetzke, T Deufel, G Hubner. Myoadenylate deaminase deficiency: successful symptomatic therapy by high dose oral administration of ribose. Klin Wochenschr 1986;64:1281-1290.

Vinpocetine

1. B. Vamosi et al (1976) "Comparative study of the effect of Ethyl Apovincaminate and Xanthinol Nicotinate in cerebrovascular diseases" Arzneim Forsch (drug research) 28, 1980-84. Hereafter abbreviated "AF (DR)")

2. F. Solti et al (1976) "Effect of Ethyl Apovincaminate on the cerebral circulation" AF(DR) 28, 1945-47.

3. E. Karpaty & L. Szporny (1976) "General and cerebral harmodynamic activity of Ethyl Apovincaminate" AF(DR)28, 1908-12.

4. Szobor and M. Klein (1976) "Ethyl Apovincaminate therapy in neurovascular

disease" AF(DR) 28, 1984-89.

5. D. Sauer et al (1988) "Vinpocetine prevents ischaemic cell damage in rat hippocampus" Life Sci. 43, 1733-39.
6. R. Branconnier (1983) "The efficacy of the cerebral metabolic enhancers in the treatment of senile dementia." Psychopharm Bull 19, 212-19.
7. Hoffer & M. Walker, Smart Nutrients, Garden City Park, NY: Avery, 1994.
8. Nicholson (1990) "Pharmacology of nootropics and metabolically active compounds in relation to their use in dementia." Psychopharm 101, 147-59.
9. K. Biro et al (1976) "Protective activity of Ethyl Apovincaminate on ischaemic anoxia of the brain" AF(DR)28, 1918-20.
10. D. Hadjiev & S. Yancheva (1976) "Rheoencephalographic and psychological studies with Ethyl Apovincaminate in cerebral vascular insufficiency" AF(DR)28, 1947-50.
11. Kaham & M. Olah (1976) "Use of Ethyl Apovincaminate in ophthalmological therapy" AF(DR)28, 1969-72. (12). H. Olpe et al (1985) "Locus Coeruleus as a target for psychogeriatric agents" Ann NY Acad Sci 444, 399-405.
12. H. Olpe et al (1985) "Locus Coeruleus as a target for psychogeriatric agents" Ann NY Acad Sci 444, 399-405.
13. B. Saletu & J. Grunberger (1985) "Memory dysfunction and vigilance; neurophysiological and psychopharmacological aspects" Ann NY Acad Sci 444, 406-27.
14. O. Ribari et al (1976) "Ethyl Apovincaminate in the treatment of sensorineuronal impairment of hearing" AF(DR)28, 1977-80.
15. R. Balestreri et al (1987) "A double blind placebo controlled evaluation of the safety and efficacy of vinpocetine in the treatment of patients with chronic vascular senile cerebral dysfunction." J. Am Geriatr Soc 35, 525-30.
16. E. Otomo et al (1985) "Comparison of vinpocetine with Ifenprodil Tartrate and Dihyroergotoxine Mesylate treatment and results of long term treatment with vinpocetine." Curr Ther Res 37, 811-21.
17. E. Cholnoky & L. Domok (1976) "Summary of safety tests of Vinpocetine" AF(DR)28, 1938-44.
18. Kiss B, Karpati E, Mechanism of action of vinpocetine, Acta Pharm Hung 1996 Sep;66(5):213-24
19. Szakall S, et al. Cerebral effects of a single dose of intravenous vinpocetine in chronic stroke patients: a PET study. J Neuroimaging 1998 Oct;8(4):197-204
20. Feigin VL, et al. Vinpocetine treatment in acute ischaemic stroke a pilot single-blind randomized clinical trial. Eur J Neurol. 2001 Jan;8(1)81-5.
21. Bonoczk P, et al, Role of sodium channel inhibition in neuroprotection: effect of vinpocetine. Brain Res Bull 2000 Oct;53(3):245-54.

Wheat Grass

1. Brown, L. 1979, Grasses and Identification Guide, Houghton Miffin
2. Womans World 3/4/97
3. Cordain L. Eaton, SB, Sebastian A, et al. Origins and Evaluation of the Western

Diet: health implications for the 21st century. American Journal Clinical Nutrition, 2005; 81(2): 341-54.

4. Schnabel, C. 1940 We're Harvesting Our Crops Too Late! Magazine Digest, November, 1940.

5. Gallagher, J., Biscoe, P., and Wallace, J. 1979. Field Studies of Cereal Leaf Growth. Journal of Experimental Botany. 30657-668.

6. Kohler, G. 1944. The effect of stages of growth on chemistry of the grasses. The Journal of Biological Chemistry 152:215-223.

7. Wigmore, Ann. The Wheatgrass Book, Avery Publishers.

8. Schnable, C. 1935. The biological value of high protein cereal grasses paper presented to the biological section of the ACS (American Chemical Society), New York April 22, 1935.

9. Bing, F. Secretary, AMA Council on Foods, 1939. Accepted foods – Cerophyll. The Journal of the American Medical Association, 112:733.

10. Graham, W., Kohler, G. and Schnable, C. 1940. "Grass As A Food: Vitamin Content". Paper presented on April 10, 1940, The American Chemical Society's 99th meeting.

11. Borasky, R. and Bradbury, J. 1942. Frozen plant juice as the source of a rabbit ovulating factor. American Journal of Physiology 137:637-639.

12. Bradbury, J. 1944. The rabbit ovulating factor of plant juice. American Journal of Physiology 142:487-493.

13. von Wendt, G. 1935. A recently discovered nutritive factor in milk. Reviewed in Kohler, G. 1953. The unidentified vitamins of grass and alfalfa. Feedstuffs, August 8, 1953.

14. Singleton, J. 1940. A measure in the treatment of menoirhagia, Kansas City Medical Journal, March, 1940

15. Colio, L. and Babb, V. 1948. Study of a new stimulatory growth factor. Journal of Biological Chemistry, 174:405-409.

16. Cheney, G. 1950. Anti-peptic ulcer dietary factor. Journal of the American Dietetic Association 26:668-672.

17. Clasen, A. 1939. Hypovitaminosis and its relationship to disease. Kansas City Medical Journal, May, 1939. P. 23.

18. Wigmore, Ann. The Wheatgrass Book.

19. Kulvinskas, V. 1976, Survival Into the Twenty-First Century, Omangod Press Wethersfield, CT

20. Cousens, M.D., Gabriel. A green path to healing and rejuvenation. Body Mind Spirit Magazine, June-July 1996.

21. Spector, H. and Calloway, D. 1959. Reduction of x-radiation mortality by cabbage and broccoli. Proceedings of the Society for Experimental Biology and Medicine 100:405-407.

22. Lai, C., Dabney, B. and Shaw, C. 1978. Inhibition of in-vitro metabolic activation of carcinogens of wheat sprout extracts. Nutrition and Cancer 1:27-30

23. Schultz, D. 1979. Sprouts vs Cancer? Checkup on medicine in: Science News. May 1979, Page 78.

24. Lai, C., Butler, M., and Matney, T. 1980. Antimutagenic activities of common

vegetables and their chlorophyll content. Mutation Research. 77:245-250.

25. Kimm, S., Tschai, B., and Park, S. 1982. Antimutagenic activity of chlorophyll to digest and indirect-acting mutagens and its contents in the vegetables. Korean Journal of Biochemistry 14:1-7.

26. Ong, T., Whang, W., Stewart, J. and Brockman, H. 1986. Chlorophyllin: a potent antimutagen against environmental and dietary complex mixtures. Mutation Research 173:111-15.

27. Perricone, N. 2004. The Perricone Promise, Warner Books.

28. Trock, B., Lanza, E. and Greenwald, P. 1990 Dietary Fiber, Vegetables and Colon Cancer: Critical Review and Meta-analysis of the Epidemiologic Evidence. Journal National Cancer Institute, 82, 650-661

29. Steinmetz, K.A. and Potter, J.D. 1996 Vegetables, Fruit and Cancer Prevention: A Review. Journal American Dietetic Association. 96, 1027-1039.

30. World Cancer Research Fund and American Institute for Cancer Research, 1997. Food, nutrition and the prevention of cancer: a global perspective Washington, D.C.: American Institute for Cancer Research.

31. Cohen, Jennifer, et al. Fruit and Vegetable Intakes and Prostate Cancer Risk. Journal of the National Cancer Institute, Vol. 92, January 5, 2000, pp.61-68.

32. Smith, L. 1955. The present status of topical chlorophyll therapy. The NY State Journal of Medicine, July 15, 1955, P. 2041-2049.

33. Gruskin, B., 1940. Chlorophyll – its therapeutic place in acute and suppurative disease. American Journal of Surgery 49:49-55.

34. Smith, L. The present status of topical chlorophyll therapy. The NY State Journal of Medicine. July 15, 1955, p. 2041-2049.

35. Journal of the National Cancer Institute, Jan. 4, 1995.

36. Davis C, et al. "Past, Present and Future of the Food Guide Pyramid" Journal American Dietetic Association 2001, 100(8):881-5

37. Dixon B. et al. "Let the Pyramid Guide Your Food Choices: Capturing the Total Diet Concept". Journal of Nutrition 2001, 131:461S-472S.

38. Dyckman, L., United States General Accounting Office, Report to Congressional Requests, July 2002, Fruits and Vegetables, Enhanced Federal Efforts to Increase Consumption Could Yield Health Benefits for Americans.

39. Ben-Arye E et al. "Wheatgrass juice in the treatment of active distal ulcerative colitis: a randomized double-blind placebo-controlled trial." Scand, J. gastroenterol, 2002, 37, 4:444-449.

40. Wigmore, A. The Hippocrates Diet and Health Program. 4:27 Avery Pub.

41. Balch, P., Balch, J., Prescription for Nutritional Healing, Third Edition, 2000, Avery Pub. 3:706

42. Womans World, 3/4/97.

43. Perricone, N. 2004, The Perricone Promise, Chapter 4, "Ten Superfoods for Age-Defying Beauty", Warner Books, NY, NY,

44. Marwaha, R. K., Bansal, D., Kaur, S., Trehan, A., Wheat Grass Juice Reduces Transfusion Requirements in Patients with Thalassemia Major: A Pilot Study. Rev. January 11, 2004.

45. Dr. Leonard Smith, Gainesville, Florida wheat grass juices.

46. Collins, K. Fight cancer with dark green vegetables, average adult should eat three cups a week. Special to MSNBC.Com April 8, 2005.
47. Healthy Eating: A Closer Look at Vegetables and Fruits, Harvard Health Pub. Boston, Mass., harvardhealth.gather.com May 27, 2008.
48. Robinson, A. 1979. Diet and Cancer in: Baron's Mailbag. Baron's Sept. 3, 1979, p. 7
49. Allison, A.C., The possible role of Vitamin K deficiency in the pathogenesis of Alzheimer's disease and in augmenting brain damage associated with cardiovascular disease. Medical Hypotheses. 2001 Aug: 57(2):151-155.
50. Sakamoto N. Wakabayashi l, Sakamoto, K. Low vitamin intake effects on glucose tolerance in rats. International Journal on Vitamin Research 1999 Jan: 69 (1): 27-31.
51. Guthrie, H. 1983 Introductory Nutrition (5th Edition). C.V. Mosby Co. St. Louis
52. Scott, M. 1986, Nutrition of Humans and Selected Animal Species. John Wiley & Sons. New York

Whey Protein

1. Blomstrand, E. and Newsholme, E.A., 1992. "Effect of branched-chain amino acid supplementation on the exercise-induced change in aromatic amino acid concentration in human muscle." Acta Physiol. Scand., 146:293-298
2. Bronner, F., 1999. "Calcium in exercise and sport." In Macroelements, Water, and Electrolytes. Eds. Driskell, J.A., and Wolinsky, J.A. CRC Press, 17-27.
3. Esmarck, J.L., Andersen, Olsen, S., Richter, E.A., Mizuno, M., and Kjaer, M., 2001, "Timing of post-exercise protein intake is important for muscle hypertrophy with resistance training in elderly humans." Journal of Physiology, 535.1:301-311.
4. Griffiths, H.R., 2000. "Antioxidants and protein oxidation." Free Radical Research, Supplement, 33:S47-58.
5. Hoerr R.A., Bostwick E.F., 2000. "Bioactive proteins and probiotic bacteria: modulators of nutritional health." Nutrition, July-August, 16(7-8): 711-713.
6. Kreider, R., Miriel, V., and Bertun, E., 1993. "Amino acid supplementation and exercise performance." Sports Medicine, 16:190-209.
7. Lemon, W.R. et al, 1996. "Is increased dietary protein necessary or beneficial for individuals with a physically active lifestyle?" Nutrition Reviews Supplement, 54: S169-175.
8. Lemon, W.R., 1998. "Effects of exercise on dietary protein requirements." International Journal of Sport Nutrition and Exercise Metabolism, 8(4): 426-447.
9. Raguso, C.A., Pereira, P., Young, V.R., 1999. "A tracer investigation of obligatory oxidative amino acid losses in healthy young adults." American Journal of Clinical Nutrition, October, 70(4):474-483.
10. Schena, F., Guerrini, F., Tregnaghi, P., and Kayser, B., 1992. "Branched-chain amino acid supplementation during trekking at high altitude." European Journal of Applied Physiology, 65:394-398.
11. Van Hall, G., Saris, W.H.M., Van De Schoor, P.A., and Watenmakers, A.J.M., 2000. "The effects of free glutamine and peptide ingestion on the rate of muscle glycogen

re-synthesis in man." International Journal of Sports Medicine, 21:25-30.

12. Yu, Y.M., Ryan C.M., Castillo L., Lu X.M., Beaumier L., Tompkins R.G., Young V.R., 2001. "Arginine and ornithine kinetics in severely burned patients: increased rate of arginine disposal." American Journal of Physiol Endocrinol Metabolism, March, 280(3):E509-E517.

13. Boirie, Y., et al., 1997. "Slow and fast dietary proteins differently modulate post-prandial protein accretion." Proceedings of the National Academy of Sciences, 94:14930-14935.

14. Dangin, M., Boirie, Y., Guillet, C., and Beaufrere, B. 2002. "Influence of the protein digestion rate on protein turnover in young and elderly subjects." Journal of Nutrition, October, 132:3228S-3233S.y of Sciences, 94:14930-14935.

15. Tolia, V., Lin, C., and Kuhns, L. 1992. "Gastric emptying using three different formulas in infants with gastroesophaegeal reflux." Journal of Pediatric Gastroenterology and Nutrition, 15(3):297-301.

16. Appel, L. et. al., 1997. "A clinical trial of the effects of dietary patterns on blood pressure." The New England Journal of Medicine, 336(16):1117-1124.

17. FitzGerald, R.J., Meisel, H., 1999. "Lactokinins: Whey protein-derived ACE inhibitory peptides." Nahrung 43:165-167.

18. FitzGerald, R.J., Meisel, H., 2000. "Milk protein-derived peptide inhibitors of angiotensin -1-converting enzyme." British Journal of Nutrition. 84:S33-S37.

19. Groziak S.M, Miller G.D., 2000. "Natural bioactive substances in milk and colostrum: effects on the arterial blood pressure system." British Journal of Nutrition, Supplement, November, 84(1):S119-S125.

20. McCarron, D.A., 1998. "Diet and high blood pressure - the paradigm shift." Science, 281:933.

21. McCarron, D. A., 2000. "Dietary calcium and blood pressure control: lessons learned from controlled clinical trials." Bulletin of the International Dairy Federation, 353:6-9.

22. Miller, G.D. et al., 2000. "Benefits of dairy product consumption on blood pressure in humans: a summary of the biomedical literature." Journal of the American College of Nutrition, April 19 (2 Suppl): S147-S164.

23. Mullally, M., Meisel, H. and Fitzgerald, R., 1997. "Angiotensin-I-Converting enzyme inhibitory activities of gastric and pancreatic proteinase digests of whey proteins." International Dairy Journal, 7:299-303.

24. Pfeuffer, M., Schrezenmeir, J., 2000. "Bioactive substances in milk with properties decreasing risk of cardiovascular diseases." British Journal of Nutrition, Supplement, 84(1):S155-S159.

25. Pihlanto-Leppala, A. et.al., 2000. "Angiotensin I-converting enzyme inhibitory properties of whey protein digest: concentration and characterization of active peptides." Journal of Dairy Research, 67:53-64.

26. Pins, J., and Keenan, J., 2002. The antihypertensive effects of a hydrolyzed whey protein isolate supplement (BioZate 1®).Cardiovascular Drugs and Therapy, 16(Supp. 1):68.

27. Rutherford, K. J., Gill, H.S., 2000. "Peptides affecting coagulation." British Journal of Nutrition, 84:S99-S102.

28. Sharpe, S.J., Gamble, G.D., Sharpe, D.N., 1994. "Cholesterol-lowering and blood pressure effect of immune milk." American Journal of Clinical Nutrition, 59:929-934.

29. Bounous, G., 2000. "Whey protein concentrate (WPC) and glutathione modulation in cancer treatment." Anticancer Research, 20:4785-4792.

30. Bounous, G., Baptist, G., and Gold, P., 1991. "Whey proteins in cancer prevention." Cancer Letters 57:91.

31. Hakkak, R., Korourian, S., Shelnutt, S. R., et. al., 2000. "Diets containing whey proteins or soy protein isolate protect against 7,12-Dimethylbenz (a) anthracene-induced mammary tumors in female rats." Cancer Epidemiology, Biomarkers & Prevention, 9:113-117.

32. Hakkak, R., Korourian, S., Ronis, M.J., Johnston, J., and Badger, T., 2001. "Dietary whey protein protects against azoxymethand-induced colon tumors in male rats." Cancer Epidemiology, Biomarkers & Prevention, 10:555-558.

33. Kennedy, R. et. al., 1995. "The use of a whey protein concentrate in the treatment of patients with metastatic carcinoma: A phase I-II clinical study." Anticancer Research, 15:2643-2650.

34. McIntosh, G.H., et al., 1995. "Dietary proteins protect against dimethylhydrazine-induced intestinal cancers in rats." Journal of Nutrition, 125:809-816.

35. Takada, Y., Aoe, S., Kumegawa, M., 1996. "Whey protein stimulates the proliferation and differentiation of osteoblastic MC3T3-E1 Cells." Biochemical and Biophysical Research Communications, 223:445-449.

36. Tsai, W., Chang, W., Chen, C.H., and Lu, F., 2000. "Enhancing effect of patented whey protein isolate (Immunocal) on the cytotoxicity of anti-cancer drug." Nutrition and Cancer, 38(2):200-208.

37. Tsuda, H., et al, 2000. "Milk and dairy products in cancer prevention: focus on bovine lactoferrin." Mutation Research, 462:227-233.

38. Bounous, G., Gervais, F., Amer, V., Batist, G., Gold, P., 1989. "The influence of dietary protein on tissue glutathione and the diseases of aging." Clinical Investigative Medicine, 12, 6:343.

39. Bounous, G, Gold, P., 1991. "The biological activity of undenatured dietary whey proteins: role of glutathione." Clinical Investigative Medicine, 14(4):296-309.

40. Bounous, G. et. al., 1989. "Immunoenhancing property of dietary whey protein in mice: role of glutathione." Clinical Investigative Medicine, 12:154-161.

41. Bounous, G., Molson, J., 1999. "Competition for glutathione precursors between the immune system and the skeletal muscle: Pathogenesis of chronic fatigue syndrome." Medical Hypothesis, 53(4):347-349.

42. Docena, G.H. et. al., 1996. "Identification of casein as the major allergenic and antigenic protein in cow's milk." Allergy, 51(6):412-416.

43. Kennedy, R.S., Bounous, G., Konok, G.P., Baruchel, S., Lee, T.D.G., 1995. "The use of a whey protein concentrate in the treatment of patients with metastatic carcinoma: A phase I-II Clinical Study." Anticancer Research, 15:2643-2650.

44. Kuwata, H. et.al., 1998. "Direct evidence of the generation in human stomach of anti-microbial peptide domain(lactoferricin) from ingested lactoferrin." Biochem. Biophys Acta, 1429:129-141.

45. LeBoucher, J. et al., 1999. "Modulation of immune response with ornithine A-ketoglutarate in burn injury: an arginine or glutamine dependency?" Nutrition, October, 15(10):773-777.

46. Wang, H., Ye, X., Ng, T.B., 2000. "First demonstration of an inhibitory activity of milk proteins against human immunodeficiency virus-1 reverse transcriptase and the effect of succinylation." Life Sciences, 67:2745-2752.

47. Wong, C.W. et al., 1997. "Effects of purified bovine whey factors on cellular immune functions in ruminants." Veterinary Immunology and Immunopathology, 56:85-96.

48. Beeh, M., Schlaak, J.F., Buhl, R., 2001. "Oral supplementation with whey proteins increases plasma glutathione levels of HIV infected patients." European Journal of Clinical Investigation, February, 31(2):171-178.

49. Berkhout, B. et al., 2002. "Characterization of the anti-HIV effects of native lactoferrin and other milk proteins and protein-derived peptides." Antiviral Research, 55:341-355.

50. Bounous, G. et. al., 1991. "Whey protein as a food supplement in HIV-seropositive individuals." Clinical Investigative Medicine, 16(3):204-209.

51. Bounous, G., 1997. "Immuno-enhancing properties of undenatured milk serum protein isolate in HIV patients." Conference Proceedings of the 2nd International Whey Conference, October 27-29, 293-305.

52. Jahoor, F. et. al., 1999. "Erythrocyte glutathione deficiency in symptom-free HIV infection is associated with decreased synthesis rate." American Journal of Physiology Ð Endocrinology and Metabolism, 276(1):E205-E211.

53. Micke, P., Beeh, K., Schlaak, J.F., and Buhl, R. 2001. "Oral supplementation with whey proteins increases plasma glutathione levels of HIV-infected patients." European Journal of Clinical Investigation. 31(2):171-178.

54. Hannan, M. et. al., 2000. "Effect of dietary protein on bone loss in elderly men and women: The Framingham Osteoporosis Study." Journal of Bone & Mineral Research, 15(12):2504-2512.

55. Jackson, K.A., Savaiano, D.A., 2001. "Lactose maldigestion, calcium intake and osteoporosis in African, Asian, and Hispanic-Americans." Journal of the American College of Nutrition, Supplement, April, 20(2):198S-207S.

56. Darling, P., Dunn, M., Sarwar, G., Brooks, S., Ball, R.O., and Pencharz, P., 1999. "Threonine kinetics in pre-term infants fed their mothers milk or formula with various ratios of whey to casein." American Journal of Clinical Nutrition, 69(1):105-114.

57. Giampietro, P., et al., 2001. "Hypoallergenicity of an extensively hydrolyzed whey formula." Pediatric Allergy and Immunology, 12(2):83-86.

58. Heine, W.E., et al., 1991. "The importance of alpha-lactoglobulin in infant nutrition." Journal of Nutrition, 121:277-283.

59. Jednak, M. et. al., 1999. "Protein meals reduce nausea and gastric slow wave dysrhythmic activity in first trimester pregnancy." American Journal of Physiology - Gastrointestinal and Liver Physiology, 227(4):G855-G861.

60. Jost, R. et. al., 1999. "Aspects of whey protein usage in infant nutrition, a brief review." International Journal of Food Science and Technology, 34:533-542.

61. Lonnerdal, B., Hernell, O., 1998. "Effects of feeding ultrahigh-temperature (UHT) treated infant formula with different protein concentrations or powdered formula, as compared to breast-feeding, on plasma amino acids, hematology, and trace element status." American Journal of Clinical Nutrition, August, 68(2):350-356.

62. Lucassen, P., et al., 2000. "Infantile colic: Crying time reduction with a whey hydrolysate: A double-blind, randomized, placebo-controlled trial." Pediatrics, 106(6):1349-1354

63. Merritt, R., Carter, M., Haight, M., Einsenberg, L., 1990. "Whey protein hydrolysate formula for infants with gastrointestinal intolerance to cow milk and soy protein in infant formulas." Journal of Pediatric Gastroenterology and Nutrition, 11:78-82.

64. Rigo, J., et al., 2001. "An infant formula free of glycomacropeptide prevents hyperthreoninemia in formula-fed preterm infants." Journal of Pediatric Gastroenterology and Nutrition, 32:127-130.

65. Beucher, S., Levenez, F., Yvon, M., and Corring, T., 1994. "Effects of gastric digestive products from casein on CCK release by intestinal cells in rats." Journal of Nutritional Biochemistry, December, Volume 5.

66. Layman, D., 2003. "The role of leucine in weight loss diets and glucose homeostasis." Journal of Nutrition, 133:252-256.

67. Layman, D. et al. 2003. "Increased Dietary Protein Modifies Glucose and Insulin Homeostasis in Adult Women during Weight Loss." Journal of Nutrition, 133: 405-410.

68. Layman, D. et al. 2003. "A Reduced Ratio of Dietary Carbohydrate to Protein Improves Body Composition and Blood Lipid Profiles during Weight Loss in Adult Women." Journal of Nutrition, 133: 411-417.

69. Zemel, M.B., 2003. "Mechanisms of Dairy Modulation of Adiposity." Journal of Nutrition, 133:252-256.

70. Markus, C.R., Olivier, B., et al., 2002. "Whey protein rich in alpha-lactalbumin increases the ratio of plasma tryptophan to the sum of the other large neutral amino acids and improves cognitive performance in stress-vulnerable subjects." American Journal of Clinical Nutrition, 75:1051-1056.

71. Meisel, H., Fitzgerald, R.J., 2000. "Opioid peptides encrypted in intact milk protein sequences". British Journal of Nutrition, 84:S27-S31.

72. Rayner, et. al., 2000. "Mitogenic whey extract stimulates wound repair activity in vitro and promotes healing of rat incisional wounds." American Journal of Physiology and Regulatory Integrative Comp. Physiology, 278:R1651-R1660.

73. Sawyer, L., Kontopidis, G., 2000. "The core lipocalin, bovine Beta-Lactoglobulin." Biochimica et Biophysica Acta, 1482:136-148.

74. Shah N.P., 2000. "Effects of milk-derived bioactives: an overview." British Journal of Nutrition, November, Supplement, 84(1):S3-S10.

75. Wu, S., Perez, M., Puyol, P., Sawyer, L. 1999. "Beta-Lactoglobulin binds palmitate within its central cavity." The Journal of Biological Chemistry, 274(1):170-174.

About the Authors

Ward W. Bond, Ph.D., is widely known from his writings, his television and radio appearances, and his lectures, as one of America's most prominent authorities on what has become a "hot" topic: the use of natural, safe supplements to combat health-related problems in the arena of health and fitness ...and potential problems associated with aging. Dr. Bond has specialized for 25 years in the area of nutritional research, and product development in the natural health industry.

Dr. Bond currently hosts the national daily television program, *Nutritional Living with Dr. Ward Bond* that airs on DirecTV and DishTV as well as other local cable networks and markets encompassing 59 million households. He has authored numerous articles on the therapeutic role of nutrients for optimum health. Dr. Bond holds a Ph.D. in holistic nutrition from Clayton College of Natural Health and studied herbal medicine from Dominion Herbal College and under the world-renowned medical herbalist David Hoffman.

Peggy Nelson is the author of *How to Create Powerful Newsletters* published by Bonus Books. She has spent most of her career life in the integrated marketing and advertising industry as a writer and director of creative services. A few of the clients she worked with include M&M Mars, National Geographic, Carnival Cruise Lines, AT&T, Garden Botanica, and Spa Atlantis.

Today she enjoys her life as a writer in the healthcare industry, working with major clients throughout the United States, and specializing in health-related topics and products. In addition, she is the proud owner and director of *The Core Energy Institute* in Fort Lauderdale, Florida. Her business focuses on Core Structural Integration and Natural Nutrition for optimum health from the inside and out.

NOTES

NOTES

NOTES

NOTES

NOTES

NOTES

NOTES

NOTES

NOTES

NOTES